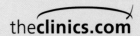

MAGNETIC RESONANCE IMAGING CLINICS

3T MR Imaging

Guest Editor

MARK C. DeLANO, MD

February 2006 • Volume 14 • Number 1

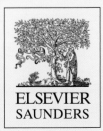

ELSEVIER SAUNDERS

An imprint of Elsevier, Inc
PHILADELPHIA LONDON TORONTO MONTREAL SYDNEY TOKYO

W.B. SAUNDERS COMPANY
A Divison of Elsevier Inc.

Elsevier Inc. • 1600 John F. Kennedy Boulevard • Suite 1800 •
Philadelphia, Pennsylvania 19103-2899

http://www.mri.theclinics.com

MRI CLINICS OF NORTH AMERICA Volume 14, Number 1
February 2006 ISSN 1064-9689, ISBN 1-4160-3530-3

Editor: Barton Dudlick

Reprints: For copies of 100 or more, of articles in this publication, please contact the Commercial
Reprints Department, Elsevier Inc., 360 Park Avenue South, New York, New York 10010-1710. Tel.
(212) 633-3813, Fax: (212) 462-1935, email: reprints@elsevier.com.

The ideas and opinions expressed in *Magnetic Resonance Imaging Clinics of North America* do not
necessarily reflect those of the Publisher. The Publisher does not assume any responsibility for
any injury and/or damage to persons or property arising out of or related to any use of the
material contained in this periodical. The reader is advised to check the appropriate medical
literature and the product information currently provided by the manufacturer of each drug to be
administered to verify the dosage, the method and duration of administration, or
contraindications. It is the responsibility of the treating physician or other health care
professional, relying on independent experience and knowledge of the patient, to determine drug
dosages and the best treatment for the patient. Mention of any product in this issue should not be
construed as endorsement by the contributors, editors, or the Publisher of the product or
manufacturers' claims.

The Magnetic Resonance Imaging Clinics of North America (ISSN 1064-9689) is published quarterly
by W.B. Saunders, 360 Park Avenue South, New York, NY 10010-1710. Months of publication are
February, May, August, and November. Business and Editorial Offices: 1600 John F. Kennedy
Boulevard, Suite 1800, Philadelphia, PA 19103-2899. Accounting and Circulation Offices: 6277
Sea Harbor Drive, Orlando, FL 32887-4800. Periodicals postage paid at New York, NY and
additional mailing offices. Subscription prices are $205.00 per year (US individuals), $305.00 per
year (US institutions), $100.00 per year (US students), $230.00 per year (Canadian individuals),
$375.00 per year (Canadian institutions), $135.00 per year (Canadian students), $280.00 per
year (international individuals), $375.00 per year (international institutions), and $135.00 per
year (international students). International air speed delivery is included in all *Clinics*
subscription prices. All prices are subject to change without notice. **POSTMASTER:** Send address
changes to *The Magnetic Resonance Imaging Clinics of North America*, Elsevier Periodicals Customer
Service, 6277 Sea Harbor Drive, Orlando, FL 32887-4800. **Customer Service: 1-800-654-2452
(US). From outside of the US, call 1-407-345-4000.**

Magnetic Resonance Imaging Clinics of North America is covered in the *RSNA Index of Imaging
Literature, Index Medicus, MEDLINE,* and *EMBASE/Excerpta Medica*.

Printed in the United States of America.

3T MR IMAGING

GUEST EDITOR

MARK C. DeLANO, MD
Associate Professor and Director of Magnetic
Resonance Imaging, Department of Radiology,
Michigan State University, East Lansing, Michigan

CONTRIBUTORS

NAFI AYGUN, MD
Assistant Professor of Radiology, The Russell H.
Morgan Department of Radiology and
Radiological Sciences, The Johns Hopkins Medical
Institution, Baltimore, Maryland

BRIAN M. DALE, PhD
Siemens Medical Solutions, Cary, North Carolina

MARK C. DeLANO, MD
Associate Professor and Director of Magnetic
Resonance Imaging, Department of Radiology,
Michigan State University, East Lansing, Michigan

J. KEVIN DeMARCO, MD
Associate Professor, Department of Radiology,
Michigan State University, East Lansing, Michigan

CHARLES FISHER
Department of Radiology, Michigan State
University, East Lansing, Michigan

JOHN HUSTON III, MD
Professor of Radiology, MR Research Lab, Mayo
Clinic, Rochester, Minnesota

ELMAR M. MERKLE, MD
Associate Professor, Department of Radiology,
Duke University Medical Center, Durham, North
Carolina

TIMOTHY J. MOSHER, MD
Associate Professor of Radiology and
Orthopaedics, Vice Chair for Clinical Radiology
Research, Chief of Musculoskeletal Imaging and

MRI, Department of Radiology, Penn State Milton
S. Hershey Medical Center, Hershey, Pennsylvania

ANDREW K. NASH, MS
Research Assistant, College of Human Medicine,
Michigan State University, East Lansing, Michigan

ERIK K. PAULSON, MD
Professor, Department of Radiology, Duke
University Medical Center, Durham, North
Carolina

R. RICHARD RAMNATH, MD
Chief of 3T Musculoskeletal, Body, and Vascular
MR Imaging, Neuroskeletal Imaging, Melbourne,
Florida

MARC D. SHAPIRO, MD
Chief of Neuroradiology, NeuroSkeletal Imaging
Institute of Winter Park, Winter Park; and
Voluntary Associate Professor of Radiology, Miller
School of Medicine, University of Miami, Miami,
Florida

LAWRENCE N. TANENBAUM, MD, FACR
Section Chief of MRI, CT, and Neuroradiology,
Edison Imaging—JFK Medical Center, New Jersey
Neuroscience Institute, Seton Hall School of
Graduate Medical Education, Edison, New Jersey

S. JAMES ZINREICH, MD
Professor of Radiology, The Russell H. Morgan
Department of Radiology and Radiological
Sciences, The Johns Hopkins Medical Institution,
Baltimore, Maryland

3T MR IMAGING

Volume 14 · Number 1 · February 2006

Contents

With appropriate adjustments to scanning protocols, one can master the challenges of scanning at 3T, and studies of the brain, spine, chest, abdomen, pelvis, vasculature, and extremities can be consistently higher in quality than those obtained at 1.5T. The greater sensitivity to magnetic susceptibility offers unique benefits in functional neuroimaging, and available software/hardware packages enhance clinical setting feasibility. The greater overall signal of 3T can be manipulated to make scanning more comfortable and with less motion artifact because scan times could be half as long.

This article illustrates the underlying physical principles of abdominal MR imaging at 3T and their impact on signal-to-noise ratio, susceptibility artifacts, chemical shift artifacts, and standing-wave effects. Abdominal MR sequence protocols also are discussed with emphasis on the sequence modifications that are required during ultrahigh-field MR imaging. Finally, basic recommendations are provided to help identify patient groups that are likely to benefit from an ultrahigh-field MR study and patient groups that probably should undergo a standard 1.5T abdominal MR examination.

As 3T MR imaging systems become more ubiquitous in the assessment of musculoskeletal disorders, an in-depth understanding of the benefits of the higher field strength is necessary to apply its added signal appropriately. This article discusses the spatial resolution and scanning speed opportunities at 3T as applied specifically to the musculoskeletal system. In addition, the various challenges that arise at higher field strengths are addressed in detail. Techniques and methods to mitigate these imaging challenges are discussed as they pertain to the musculoskeletal system. An overview of currently available 3T extremity coils also is provided.

3T MR Imaging of the Musculoskeletal System (Part II): Clinical Applications 41

R. Richard Ramnath

The clinical application of 3T MR imaging in the musculoskeletal system has vast and exciting potential. Although the overall diagnostic ability on 1.5T systems is excellent, many areas need definite improvement. There are several specific anatomic structures in each of the six major joints that generally are evaluated suboptimally on conventional field strengths. These areas of deficiency possess the greatest potential for demonstrating the advantages of higher field strength systems. By exploiting the added signal-to-noise ratio, the higher spatial resolution, and the increased contrast-to-noise ratio of the intrinsic structures of joints, radiologists are poised to make dramatic headway in the diagnostic capabilities of MR imaging in the musculoskeletal system.

Musculoskeletal Imaging at 3T: Current Techniques and Future Applications 63

Timothy J. Mosher

This article reviews techniques for optimizing 3T musculoskeletal (MSK) MR imaging along with methods for minimizing image artifact. Current clinical experience with standard MR imaging protocols are reviewed and illustrated with case examples. Finally, emerging applications of ultrahigh-field MSK MR imaging is presented.

3T MR Imaging of the Brain 77

Mark C. DeLano and Charles Fisher

The clinical applications of 3T MR imaging in the central nervous system have been evolving rapidly since the US Food and Drug Administration approved higher field strength for clinical practice in 1998. Although most challenges that initially limited the dissemination and adoption of 3T MR devices have been addressed, the full potential of the added value of high field is dependent on the choices that are made in protocol implementation and hardware development. As with the transitions between low and high field, proper field-specific parameter selection remains critical for the establishment of clinical protocols at 3T. Each pulse sequence requires field-specific modifications. This article discusses the issues of 3T clinical protocol development for brain imaging and demonstrates methods to achieve the greatest potential of higher field strength systems.

Head and Neck Imaging at 3T 89

Nafi Aygun and S. James Zinreich

In the past decades significant advances in imaging with 1.5T units have benefited head and neck imaging. It is hoped that the 3T units, now commercially available, will provide an exponential advance in the evaluation of this body part. This article aims to justify our expectations based on physical principles. A discussion of the advantages and disadvantages of head and neck imaging at 3T in our experience and those of others is provided.

MR Imaging of the Spine at 3T

Marc D. Shapiro

Many advantages and challenges are associated with 3T imaging of the spine. The increase in signal-to-noise ratio allows for optimization of diagnostic quality and improved clinical efficiency. Parallel imaging techniques merge well with high-field technology, which minimizes many of the challenges that are associated with 3T systems. The increase in chemical shift, pulsatile flow, and susceptibility artifact can be mediated with manipulation of imaging parameters. Despite the challenges, 3T imaging of the spine provides many improvements over 1.5T systems, and with developing technology and pulse sequence design, the improvements can be maximized.

Extracranial Carotid MR Imaging at 3T

J. Kevin DeMarco, John Huston III, and Andrew K. Nash

This article reviews current controversy involving the accuracy of 1.5T contrast-enhanced MR angiography to depict carotid stenosis and the potential implication for improved extracranial carotid MR angiography with 3T MR scanners. In addition to using 8-channel neurovascular coils to image the entire course of the carotid arteries from the aortic through the circle of Willis with 3T MR scanners, the potential of even higher resolution carotid bifurcation MR angiography and *in vivo* carotid plaque imaging with dedicated surface coils at 3T also is discussed.

Index

FORTHCOMING ISSUES

May 2006

Breast MR Imaging

Christiane Kuhl, MD, *Guest Editor*

August 2006

MR Imaging of Cartilage

Philipp Lang, MD, *Guest Editor*

RECENT ISSUES

November 2005

MR Imaging of the Hip

Zehava Sadka Rosenberg, MD, *Guest Editor*

August 2005

MR-Guided Interventions

Jonathan S. Lewin, MD, *Guest Editor*

GOAL STATEMENT

The goal of *Magnetic Resonance Imaging Clinics of North America* is to keep practicing radiologists and radiology residents up to date with current clinical practice in radiology by providing timely articles reviewing the state of the art in patient care.

ACCREDITATION

The *Magnetic Resonance Imaging Clinics of North America* is planned and implemented in accordance with the Essential Areas and Policies of the Accreditation Council for Continuing Medical Education (ACCME) through the joint sponsorship of the University of Virginia School of Medicine and Elsevier. The University of Virginia School of Medicine is accredited by the ACCME to provide continuing medical education for physicians.

The University of Virginia School of Medicine designates this educational activity for a maximum of 60 category 1 credits per year, 15 category 1 credits per issue, toward the AMA Physician's Recognition Award. Each physician should claim only those credits that he/she actually spent in the activity.

The American Medical Association has determined that physicians not licensed in the US who participate in this CME activity are eligible for AMA PRA category 1 credit.

Category 1 credit can be earned by reading the text material, taking the CME examination online at http://www.theclinics.com/home/cme, and completing the evaluation. After taking the test, you will be required to review any and all incorrect answers. Following completion of the test and evaluation, your credit will be awarded and you may print your certificate.

FACULTY DISCLOSURE/CONFLICT OF INTEREST

The University of Virginia School of Medicine, as an ACCME accredited provider, endorses and strives to comply with the Accreditation Council for Continuing Medical Education (ACCME) Standards of Commercial Support, Commonwealth of Virginia statutes, University of Virginia policies and procedures, and associated federal and private regulations and guidelines on the need for disclosure and monitoring of proprietary and financial interests that may affect the scientific integrity and balance of content delivered in continuing medical education activities under our auspices.

The University of Virginia School of Medicine requires that all CME activities accredited through this institution be developed independently and be scientifically rigorous, balanced and objective in the presentation/discussion of its content, theories and practices.

All authors/editors participating in an accredited CME activity are expected to disclose to the readers relevant financial relationships with commercial entities occurring within the past 12 months (such as grants or research support, employee, consultant, stock holder, member of speakers bureau, etc.). The University of Virginia School of Medicine will employ appropriate mechanisms to resolve potential conflicts of interest to maintain the standards of fair and balanced education to the reader. Questions about specific strategies can be directed to the Office of Continuing Medical Education, University of Virginia School of Medicine, Charlottesville, Virginia.

The authors/editors listed below have identified no financial or professional relationships for themselves or their spouses/partners:
Nafi Aygun, MD; J. Kevin DeMarco, MD; Barton Dudlick, Acquisitions Editor; Charles Fisher, Research Assistant; John Houston III, MD; Elmar M. Merckle, MD; Timothy J. Mosher, MD; Andrew Nash, MS; Erik K. Paulson, MD; and R. Richard Ramnath, MD.

The author listed below has identified the following professional/financial relationships for himself:
Brian M. Dale, PhD, is employed by Siemens Medical Solutions USA, Inc.

Mark C. DeLano, MD, is on the speaker's bureau for GE Healthcare.
Marc D. Shapiro, MD, is a consultant and on the speaker's bureau for GE Healthcare.
Lawrence N. Tanenbaum, MD, FACR, is on the speaker's bureau for GE Healthcare.
S. James Zinreich, MD, has stock in IZI Medical Products.

Disclosure of discussion of non-FDA approved uses for pharmaceutical and/or medical devices:
The University of Virginia School of Medicine, as an ACCME provider, requires that all authors identify and disclose any "off label" uses for pharmaceutical and medical device products. The University of Virginia School of Medicine recommends that each physician fully review all the available data on new products or procedures prior to clinical use.

TO ENROLL

To enroll in the *Magnetic Resonance Imaging Clinics of North America* Continuing Medical Education program, call customer service at 1-800-654-2452 or visit us online at http://www.theclinics.com/home/cme. The CME program is available to subscribers for an additional fee of $175.00.

MAGNETIC
RESONANCE
IMAGING CLINICS

Magn Reson Imaging Clin N Am (2006) xi

Dedication

I dedicate this issue to my wife Teri DeLano for her patience, encouragement, and continued support.

Mark C. DeLano, MD
Department of Radiology
Michigan State University
184 Radiology Building
East Lansing MI 48824-1313, USA

E-mail address: mcd@rad.msu.edu

doi:10.1016/j.mric.2006.02.002

ELSEVIER
SAUNDERS

MAGNETIC
RESONANCE
IMAGING CLINICS

Magn Reson Imaging Clin N Am (2006) xiii

Preface
3T MR Imaging

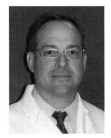

Mark C. DeLano, MD
Department of Radiology
Michigan State University
184 Radiology Building
East Lansing, MI 48824-1313, USA

E-mail address:
mcd@rad.msu.edu

Mark C. DeLano, MD
Guest Editor

The intent of this issue of the *Magnetic Resonance Imaging Clinics of North America* is to provide an overview of the recent advancements in MR imaging related to the clinical implementation of 3-Tesla (T) field strength scanners. Since its inception, MR imaging has offered progressively more detailed and accurate anatomic images and increasingly physiologic information. Ongoing technical refinements in the implementation of progressively higher-field strength instruments continue to enhance the capability of MR imaging technology to delineate human structure and function. The optimal field strength for MR imaging has been a moving target. It was thought to be 0.3T in the early 1980s and has obviously changed during the maturation of the technology. As experience was gained and solutions to the challenges of increasing field strength were devised, the subsequent literature gave support to 1.5T devices. The acceptance of 3T units likewise is growing.

The appeal of methods to increase the available signal has been universal. Many require additional scan time. Increasing the field strength provides signal without this additional burden. The advent of 3T scanners coincides with important coil and signal detection advancements in the form of parallel imaging, providing a unique synergy and opportunity to advance our capabilities to impact patient care through better imaging.

I am fortunate to have had the commitment of a number of colleague contributors, all of whom were chosen as clinicians and scientists involved in the early adoption of 3T scanners in their practice. This issue begins with a comprehensive overview of the fundamental principles of imaging at 3T with clinical examples of these principles in practice. This is followed by reviews detailing abdominal, musculoskeletal, and neuroradiologic imaging issues and their management, with clear delineation of the advantages and limitations of this imaging technique. The final article describes the application of 3T MR imaging to the problem of carotid atherosclerosis, its detection and characterization, and the potential for guiding the management of the disease.

I wish to thank all of the authors for their invaluable contributions. I hope that you will find the articles in this issue informative and provocative. I would also like to thank Barton Dudlick of Elsevier for his helpful and professional guidance in assembling this issue.

doi:10.1016/j.mric.2006.02.001

MAGNETIC
RESONANCE
IMAGING CLINICS

Magn Reson Imaging Clin N Am (2006) 1–15

Clinical 3T MR Imaging: Mastering the Challenges

Lawrence N. Tanenbaum MD, FACR

- ■ Specific absorption rate
- ■ Ambient noise
- ■ Dielectric effects
- ■ Susceptibility issues
- ■ Chemical shift effects
- ■ Tissue contrast issues
- ■ Diffusion imaging
- ■ Blood oxygenation level–dependent contrast studies
- ■ Time-of-flight neuro-MR angiography

- ■ MR spectroscopy
- ■ Body imaging
- ■ Body vascular
- ■ Musculoskeletal imaging
  Spine
  Joint imaging
- ■ Clinical practice impact
- ■ Summary
- ■ References

MR scanning began to make an impact in the clinical practice setting in the mid-1970s. At introduction, the most common systems operated at a field strength of 0.6T and there was credible doubt that more powerful magnets would be feasible, particularly for whole-body (beyond the brain) imaging needs. Technological advances made high-field MR imaging practical, and systems operating at 1.5T are the current clinical benchmark. New systems that are sold today at lower field strengths are open designs that are directed to larger or claustrophobic patients. Although there once was a significant market for closed systems operating at 1T because of the lower cost, the decreasing cost differential with 1.5T and competitive market demands have eliminated these systems from new purchase considerations.

Over the last several years, systems that operate at higher field strengths have become more prevalent, particularly at academic and research centers. An informal survey of the market at present (mid-2005) reveals that approximately 350 to 400 3T

whole-body capable MR systems are operational, with a declining 25% used primarily for research. Market projections are that about 400 new 3T systems will be installed over the next 12 months with approximately 90% planned for routine clinical setting whole-body application. Fueling the shift in interest from 1.5T to 3T and from academic to clinical practice is the validation that was once considered very high-field MR imaging (3T) is now feasible, and is potentially superior to 1.5T for clinical indications throughout the body.

At the author's clinical practice site, 3T has been used for whole-body imaging in the community setting for approximately 4 years; during the last 25 months, a third-generation, broadband 8- to 16-channel short-bore magnet system has been used. The easily recognized boost in image quality and consistency that are achieved through higher resolution and higher net signal-to-noise ratio (SNR) scanning drives referrals in all subspecialty areas. Although physicians who are engaged in the practice of neurology and neurosurgery are the first

MRI, CT, and Neuroradiology, Edison Imaging—JFK Medical Center, New Jersey Neuroscience Institute, Seton Hall School of Graduate Medical Education, 65 James Street, Edison, NJ 08818, USA
E-mail address: NuroMRI@aol.com

1064-9689/06/$ – see front matter © 2006 Elsevier Inc. All rights reserved.
mri.theclinics.com
doi:10.1016/j.mric.2005.12.004

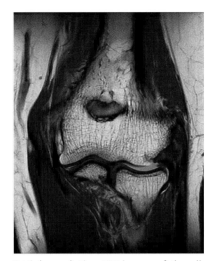

Figure 1 High resolution FSE image of the elbow.

to become aware of the benefits of 3T MR imaging and most readily direct cases to the higher field system, specialists in orthopedics, vascular surgery, and oncology rapidly follow to demand the higher overall quality of 3T (Fig. 1) [1,2].

3T MR imaging has inherent advantages over more commonly used 1.5T systems as well as some challenges that must be met for higher field MR imaging to be clinically practical. Concerns over surface coil availability, radiofrequency (RF) deposition limits, and higher ambient noise have to be addressed. Challenges with respect to system homogeneity, increased sensitivity to magnetic susceptibility and chemical shift effects, and reduced tissue contrast need to be overcome. Siting concerns differ from those of 1.5T systems because the magnets are much heavier, although the footprint and fringe field on modern systems differ only slightly from those of 1.5T systems. The final obstacle to increased penetration of 3T into the clinical setting worldwide is clear demonstration of the incremental benefits of 3T over 1.5T, with respect to image quality and efficiency (Fig. 2).

Specific absorption rate

Specific absorption rate (SAR) is a measure of energy deposited by an RF field in a given mass of tissue. SAR is limited by the International Electrotechnical Commission (IEC) not to exceed 8 W/kg of tissue for any 5-minute period or 4 W/kg for a whole body averaged over 15 minutes [3].

Dissipation of RF energy in the body can result in tissue heating. The doubling of field from 1.5T to 3.0Tleads to a quadrupling of SAR (Fig. 3). Therefore, SAR considerations inherently limit scanner performance by limiting the rate of RF energy

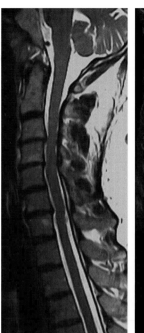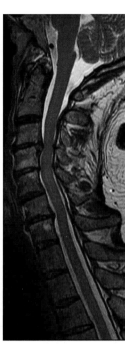

Figure 2 Comparison of 1.5T and 3T. Note the higher resolution image at 3T (*right*) in ~1/3 less scan time.

deposition and cumulative deposition to comply with SAR limitations set forth by the IEC. This can manifest as a reduction in slices per repetition time (TR), longer scan times, and "cooling" delays between acquisitions.

Manipulations that traditionally are used to limit SAR include reducing acquisition flip angle (eg, from 180° with fast spin echo [FSE] and ~40° with gradient recalled echo [GRE]) which could affect image contrast. The reduction from a flip angle of 180° (to typically ~120°) has been tolerated well thus far, without any noticeable deleterious effect on image contrast. Reducing the flip angle from what might be ideal for a contrast-enhanced three-dimensional (3D) GRE MR angiography (MRA) study (~40°), to what will deliver the shortest TR and echo time (TE) at the scanner (~25°), also is tolerated well.

Duty cycle can be defined for this purpose as the individual tasks (RF pulses) that play out during a given MR experiment (TR period). The RF energy

$$SAR \propto B^2\alpha^2D$$

B = field strength
α = flip angle
D = duty cycle

Figure 3 Specific absorption rate considerations.

that is deposited during a given scan is proportional to the intensity of the duty cycle. Longer echo train (ET) acquisitions, which are common with high-performance gradient systems and fat suppression techniques that are used commonly, particularly with musculoskeletal and body imaging, exacerbate duty cycle load. Reducing duty cycle, by using a slightly longer TR than the minimum necessary (building in cooling time, in a sense), is an effective technique that comes at the expense of only slightly longer scan times (Fig. 4).

Parallel imaging (PI) is another powerful method of reducing RF exposure and scan times by reducing the number of phase-encoding steps that is performed in a given scan. The typical trade-off in SNR (a PI factor of 2 reduces SNR by 40%) is balanced by the higher signal of 3T, and is facilitated by the improved higher SNR high-density 8- to 16-channel surface coils that are available (Fig. 5). PI is only practical for applications in which there is ample SNR at a single scan repetition (1 nex), and is most useful for applications, such as contrast-enhanced MRA and breath-hold body and cardiac imaging. As surface coil and scanning technology advances with further optimization for PI, this technique may become increasingly important at 3T [4].

Another technique for managing RF deposition load is to interleave SAR-intensive sequences with low-RF deposition scans (eg, follow a long ET, fat-suppressed FSE scan with a two-dimensional [2D] gradient echo acquisition before staring the next FSE scan; Fig. 6). This technique has limited applicability for most applications, but has some usefulness, particularly for body imaging on early-generation 3T systems.

Innovative methods of reducing SAR without imaging compromise are or will soon be available. New short-bore magnet designs—widely present

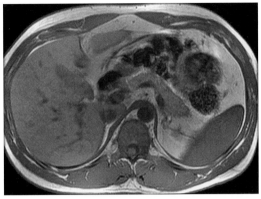

Figure 5 6-mm single breathhold in-phase gradient echo image of the liver benefits from parallel imaging techniques.

in the clinical setting—are inherently more SAR efficient than are earlier generation long-bore systems, because less of the body is exposed to the shorter transmitting body coil. Innovations in RF chain technology also have improved the efficiency of energy deposition with a resultant formidable net reduction in SAR.

Innovative pulse sequence manipulations, such as applying magnetization transfer prepulses only at the center one third of k-space, can maintain improved tissue contrast while depositing considerably less RF energy. Advances in pulse sequence design, such as reshaping RF and gradient waveforms (eg, variable rate selective excitation [VERSE] technique), reduce peak RF power up to 40% to 60% compared with conventional techniques (Fig. 7). This modification in pulse sequence design, along with others from scanner manufacturers (smooth transitions between pseudo steady stases [TRAPS], hyperechoes), also should lead to RF limitations and slice acquisition efficiency that are

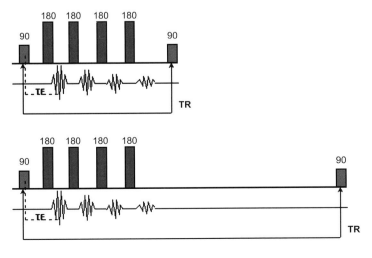

Figure 4 Doubling TR, absent other changes in the number of slices or ET, reduces the SAR by 1/2.

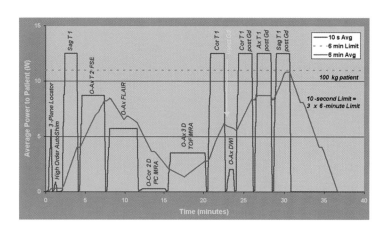

Figure 6 RF power history for 30-minute 3T clinical brain exam.

equal to or slightly greater than those that are in place at 1.5T.

Removing the body coil from the transmission process by the use of transmit-receive (T/R) surface coils has a formidable impact on RF deposition. The development and availability of an increasing number of local T/R surface coils will facilitate efficiency and encourage even higher resolution scanning by reducing the obstacle that SAR limitation presents.

Ambient noise

Sound pressure levels (SPL) increase with field strength. The noise levels at 3.0Tapproach twice that of 1.5T and can be in excess of 130 dB [5] (the IEC and the US Food and Drug Administration limit permissible sound levels to 99 dB). Higher gradient performance comes at the cost of higher SPL. The inherent noise dampening effect of magnet length and weight also influence ambient SPL; thus, the shorter bore systems that are sold today are inherently louder.

Methods of reducing SPL include passive approaches, such as the routine use of earplugs and active noise cancellation by way of headphones.

Reducing gradient performance for certain demanding applications (echoplanar imaging, balanced steady-state free precession imaging) is another approach, but this, by nature, limits clinical efficacy. Some late-generation 3T systems are equipped with advances, such as acoustically shielded vacuum-based bore liners, which keep noise levels below limits without restricting gradient performance.

Dielectric effects

Inhomogeneous RF distribution is caused by a variety of conductive and dielectric effects in tissue. Although present at 1.5T, these effects are exacerbated at higher field strength and typically manifest as image nonuniformity. The use of high SNR surface coils may increase the conspicuity of these effects for body applications, which manifest as areas of shading or signal drop-off [6].

Use of pads filled with a medium of high electric permittivity can homogenize significantly the magnetic field (B1)-distribution in tissue with high conductivity (Fig. 8). These same effects manifest as brightness in the center of the brain on studies of the head. It is a fortuitous result of the use of small

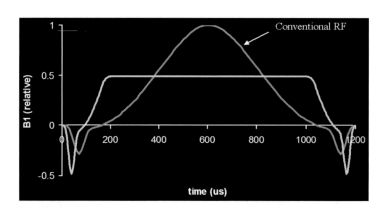

Figure 7 Pulse sequence changes such as VERSE reduce SAR without impacting contrast resolution.

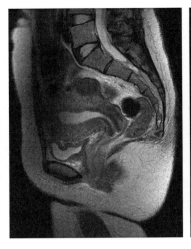 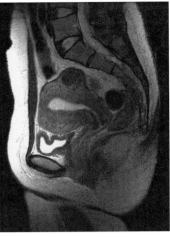

Figure 8 Dielectric effects. Note the prominent shading of the anterior abdominal wall (*left*) ameliorated with the use of a high conductivity material filled pad (*right*).

element, high-density head coils, which are brighter in the near field, that the resultant images of the brain are, in the end, highly uniform (Fig. 9).

Susceptibility issues

Susceptibility effects scale with field strength. This effect is exploited at 3T in improving the sensitivity of FSE imaging to the presence of hemorrhage and mineralization [7]. Although susceptibility effects might be expected to be prohibitive and limiting for patients with implanted hardware, appropriately designed protocols, which leverage the combination of efficient coil designs and high bandwidth scanning, keep artifact manageable and similar in severity to that of 1.5T (Fig. 10). Protocol manipulations that manage susceptibility artifact include shorter TEs, reductions in voxel size, and higher receiver bandwidth than would be used at 1.5T. The higher SNR that is afforded by 3T also permits compensation with PI in echoplanar imaging (EPI) and longer ETs with FSE acquisitions.

Susceptibility contrast–based, first-pass, gadolinium contrast–dependent perfusion imaging at 3T is plagued by signal loss in regions that are prone to susceptibility artifact, such as the frontal sinuses and skull base. Protocols that use minimum TE GRE or moderate TE spin echo (SE) acquisitions go a long way toward ameliorating these effects (Fig. 11). In addition, PI techniques reduce susceptibility artifact and distortion on single-shot EPI studies [8].

Chemical shift effects

Chemical shift effects also scale with field. This provides a boost in metabolite peak separation/resolution for spectroscopy, and makes RF fat suppression more robust at 3T than at lower field strengths. An increase in chemical shift artifact at 3T could be a significant limiting factor in routine anatomic imaging. With appropriate scanning protocols, the SNR of 3T and late-generation multichannel coils are leveraged by way of the routine use of higher

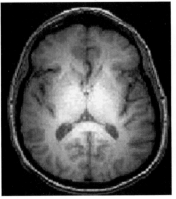 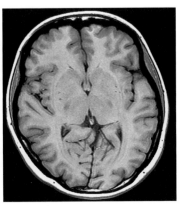

Figure 9 Note the central brightness due to dielectric effects at 3T. Images with phased array surface coils that are brighter in the near field (*left*) produce an image that is uniform at 3T.

T/R head coil   8 channel head coil

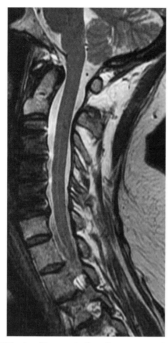

Figure 10 Study after anterior decompression, fusion, and instrumentation. High bandwidth techniques facilitated by the combination of 3T signal and a high SNR 8-channel spine coil effectively manage susceptibility artifact.

bandwidths (32–125 kHz) for SE and FSE imaging, which keeps chemical shift effects in a range similar to that of 1.5T (Fig. 12).

Tissue contrast issues

T1 (longitudinal relaxation time) relaxation times are prolonged at 3T with respect to 1.5T, which has

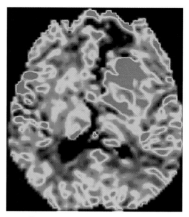

Figure 11 Perfusion image of a meningioma.

been exploited to produce superior time-of-flight (TOF) MRA studies. The same effect leads to reduced, and thus, unsatisfactory contrast resolution on traditional (short TR short TE) SE acquisitions. These considerations do not plague other methods for obtaining T1 contrast that are used widely at 1.5T, such as RF spoiled gradient recalled, magnetization-prepared techniques (eg, inversion recovery [IR] or magnetization transfer 3D SPGR [spoiled gradient recalled]) (Fig. 13).

IR techniques that produce superior T1 contrast at 1.5T, such as phase-sensitive IR for the brain (Fig. 14) and T1 fluid attenuated inversion recovery (FLAIR) for the brain, spine, and musculoskeletal system, are equally well suited to higher field imaging and can yield spectacular results (Fig. 15).

With PI techniques, T1 studies are net faster and higher in resolution than are those that are obtained at 1.5T. A routine shift to high bandwidth—moderate ET inversion recovery FSE (T1 FLAIR)—from SE

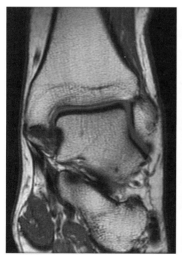
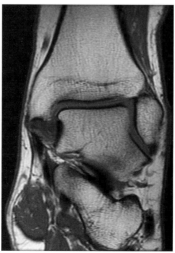

16 KHz   *32 KHz*

Figure 12 Note the severe chemical shift artifact at 16 kHz widening the appearance of the cortex of the talar dome and the expected appearance at 32 kHz.

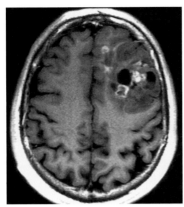

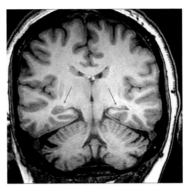

Figure 13 Residual low grade glioma. Twenty slices at 20 FOV, 288 × 192, 5-mm thick in 54 seconds with a parallel imaging acceleration factor of 2.

Figure 15 1.5-mm 3D IR SPGR study demonstrates left hippocampal atrophy.

has the additional benefit of reducing susceptibility artifact—a benefit in patients who have had surgery or who have metal implants—and chemical shift effect sensitivity (Fig. 16).

Although the relaxivity properties of gadolinium are not significantly different at 1.5T than at 3T, the longer T1 of tissues 2and higher net SNR at 3T contribute to an increase in conspicuity of enhancement (greater contrast to background ratio). Therefore, many sites use a lower dose of contrast (0.05 mmol/kg) for routine brain imaging purposes (Fig. 17).

T2 (transverse relaxation time) values in biologic tissues are unchanged or are decreased only slightly with increases in field strength. T2* effects scale with field strength, and thus, 3T studies are more sensitive to deposition of blood products and tissue mineralization.

Diffusion imaging

The greater signal intensity that is afforded at 3T is particularly enticing for diffusion weighted imaging

(DWI) needs. SNR can be marginal for routine clinical imaging purposes at 1.5T, and the quest for higher B values (>1000 s/mm^2), thinner slices (<3 mm), and white matter anisotropy mapping (tensor imaging) further stresses the SNR equation (Fig. 18) [9].

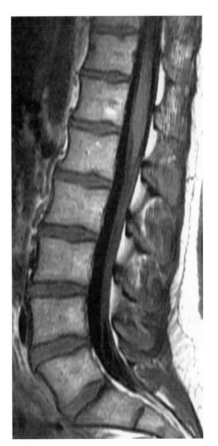

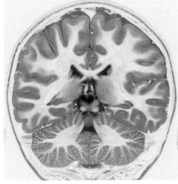

Figure 14 3-mm phase sensitive inversion recovery studies create dramatic T1 contrast.

Figure 16 T1 FLAIR study obtained in an 8-channel spine coil. Note the excellent T1 contrast and absence of significant chemical shift artifact.

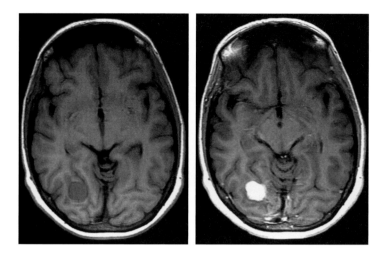

Figure 17 Pre- (*left*) and post-2.5 cc gadobenate dimeglumine images of the brain of a meningioma (T1 FLAIR).

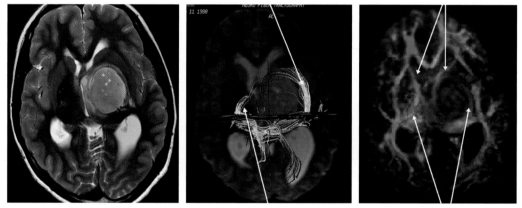

Figure 18 Tensor DWI tractography identifies posterior and lateral displacement of motor fibers (*blue*) within the posterior limb of the internal capsule leading to resection from a medial approach. No motor defecit was present after surgery.

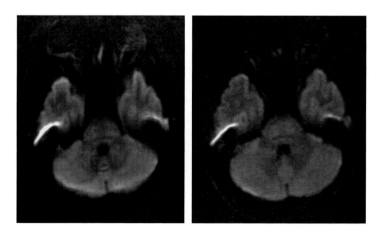

Figure 19 Note reduced distortion with ASSET (*right*). Distortion due to susceptibility artifact is proportional to field strength.

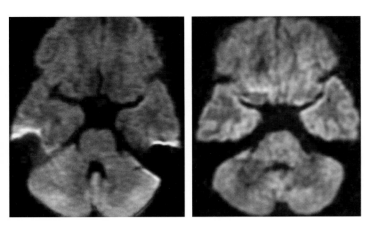

Figure 20 Comparison of EPI (*left*) and PROPELLER FSE DWI. Note significantly less distortion with FSE.

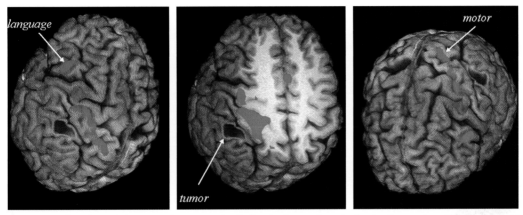

Figure 21 Superior views. Motor study proves the lesion is situated posterior to the postcentral gyrus and thus resectable. Note ipsilateral hemispheric language dominance.

DWI studies at high field strength typically are acquired by using EPI techniques. These single-shot studies are inherently prone to susceptibility artifact, which can limit evaluation of structures in close proximity to the bony skull base and air-filled paranasal sinuses. The artifact is exacerbated by the presence of metal (eg, from dentures, dental braces, foreign bodies). Because susceptibility scales with field strength, these artifacts are proportionally worse at higher field strengths. PI techniques are applied routinely on modern 3T systems that are equipped with optimized surface coils and broadband reconstruction hardware, which effectively balances these considerations by decreasing the echo spacing and TE of the scan. This reduces susceptibility artifact and ameliorates signal loss that is due to T2 decay on these long-ET acquisitions (Fig. 19).

Multishot FSE DWI techniques (eg, propeller), which are inherently less sensitive to susceptibility, have increased usefulness as a result at 3T (Fig. 20) [10].

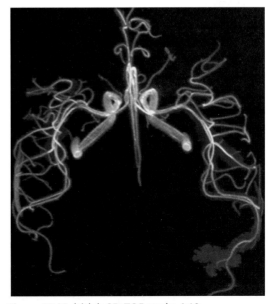

Figure 22 Multislab 3D TOF study, 4:10.

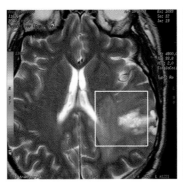
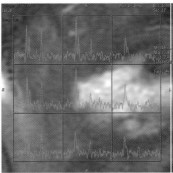

Figure 23 Differentiation of radiation necrosis from recurrent tumor. 2D chemical shift imaging study reveals a striking elevation of choline metabolites consistent with viable tumor.

Blood oxygenation level–dependent contrast studies

Perhaps the greatest impact of 3T in neuroimaging is in the enhanced quality and consistency of blood oxygenation level–dependent contrast (BOLD) functional imaging. The greater susceptibility contrast sensitivity and higher SNR that are inherent to 3T scanning can produce up to a 40% increase in detected activation with BOLD imaging, over 1.5T (Fig. 21) [11]. Improved contrast resolution enhances the success rate of these procedures for routine presurgical mapping of eloquent cortex (eg, sensorimotor, language), and coupled with scanner-integrated paradigm delivery, have facilitated community practice use to evaluate diseases, such as dementia and other psychiatric disorders.

Time-of-flight neuro-MR angiography

The longer T1 of background tissues can be exploited for superior inflow MRA (TOF MRA). Scanning techniques use lower flip angles, which manages RF deposition and reduces pulsation artifacts. The higher SNR that is provided by 3T with eight-channel surface coils encourages the routine use of high imaging matrices (512–1024) and produces studies that can rival the resolution of catheter angiography (DSA [digital subtraction angiography]) (Fig. 22) [12,13]. Optimized coils, coupled with PI techniques, maintain scan times that are similar to or shorter than those at 1.5T.

MR spectroscopy

Chemical shift doubles when moving from 1.5T to 3T and results in improved spectral resolution. This may allow routine evaluation of metabolites that may be obscured at 1.5T [14]. Along with the higher SNR of 3T, this may increase the efficacy of proton and multinuclear spectroscopy of many disorders (Fig. 23).

Body imaging

RF deposition limits the number of slices that is available per given time, which encourages multiple breath hold acquisitions, particularly with 2D GRE. Optimized 3D GRE acquisitions benefit from the high SNR of 3T and high-density coils to produce thin slice, functionally isotropic volumetric whole

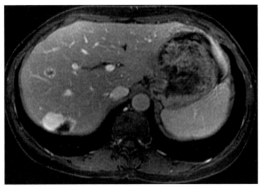

Figure 24 3D GRE fat suppressed 3-mm hepatic phase image reveals two right lobe hepatic hemangiomas.

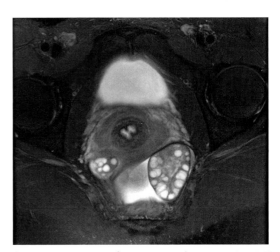

Figure 25 20-cm FOV fat suppressed 7-mm 512 × 512 study.

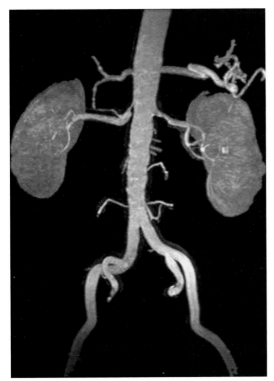

Figure 26 High resolution renal MRA study obtained with 0.1 mmol/kg of gadolinium. Study obtained with a 35-cm FOV and 2-mm partitions every 1 mm.

abdominal scans in a single breath hold (Fig. 24). Motion-resistant techniques with single-shot FSE and respiratory-triggered multishot FSE also are used commonly. Eight-channel phased-array surface coil designs that are optimized for PI ameliorate many SAR-based restrictions.

Studies of the abdomen and pelvis are accomplished routinely with thinner slices and higher imaging matrices—comparable to those that are used with CT—which facilitates comparison and lesion characterization (see Fig. 24; Fig. 25) [15]. The higher SNR that is afforded by 3T also may facilitate applications (eg, spectroscopy) and might obviate the need for endocavitary surface coils for advanced applications (eg, prostate imaging) (see Fig. 25).

Body vascular

The higher SNR of 3T, coupled with PI-compatible surface coils, produce high-quality, higher spatial resolution, contrast-enhanced vascular studies with greater consistency than at 1.5T [16]. Decreasing the flip angle reduces SAR, and as a result, keeps TE and TR in a range similar to that of 1.5T. The longer T1 values of background tissues augments the visualization of intravascular contrast and

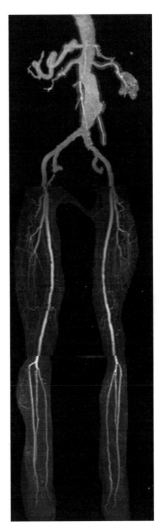

Figure 27 3T runoff study. Time resolved imaging with time resolved imaging of contrast kinetics (TRICKS) protocol is used for lower two stations. The final of three acquisitions is a high resolution single phase acquisition.

potentially allows a reduction in the contrast dose that is administered (Fig. 26). Although full-body vascular coils are not available, the increasing importance of multistation time-resolved MRA techniques at the expense of so-called "bolus-chasing" reduces their significance (Fig. 27). Dedicated high-density coil designs, such as a "boot" coil, should allow image quality that is unattainable at 1.5T.

Musculoskeletal imaging

Spine

Eight-channel phased-array coils are widely available for spine imaging. Practical considerations

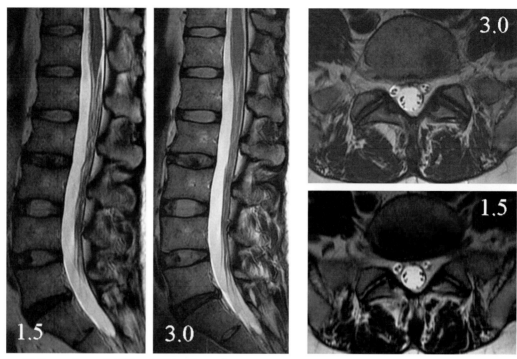

Figure 28 Comparison of 1.5T and 3T lumbar spine.

yield studies that are more consistent in quality at higher resolution and are about one third faster than those of 1.5T (Fig. 28) [17]. Although susceptibility is a theoretic concern, long ET high-bandwidth acquisitions yield excellent image quality, even for patients with implanted metal hardware. Further testing is required before the safety of spine-implanted electronic devices can be established fully.

Joint imaging

Responsible for more than 20% of the study volume of the typical clinical scanner, the quality of joint imaging is a major factor in determining the financial feasibility of higher field MR imaging. Coil availability has been limited until recently, and SAR concerns are prominent because high duty cycle applications (eg, fat suppression, long ET FSE) are common. The homogeneity of the latest generation short-bore devices is critical because joints rarely are scanned near the isocenter, and fat suppression is important to maintain contrast resolution (Fig. 29).

High-quality, high SNR, phased-array surface coils are becoming available, and generally provide studies that are recognizably superior to those from

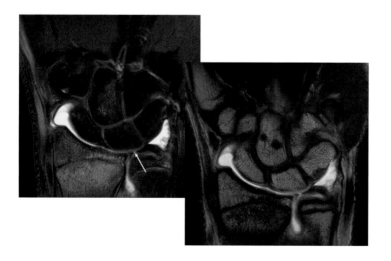

Figure 29 Postarthrographic study demonstrating a tear of the triangular fibrocartilage complex. RF fat sat T2 (*left*), T1 SE (*right*). 3-mm slices, 8-cm FOV 512 matrix.

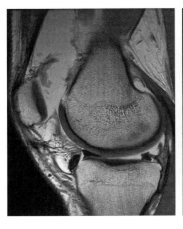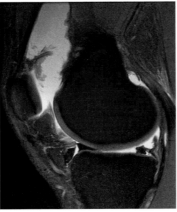

Figure 30 8-channel phased array (In Vivo Corporation) knee images demonstrate a displaced meniscal tear.

1.5T systems, often in significantly less time (Fig. 30). Offering higher spatial resolution, 3T MR imaging may yield additional information that is useful in the study of smaller parts and cartilage than do examinations that are obtained at 1.5T. Studies that are obtained with older and less capable coils (eg, quadrature) benefit from the SNR of 3T to be competitive with studies that are obtained with more advanced surface coils at 1.5T.

Receive-only coils require SAR-intensive body coil transmission, which limits performance. The increasing availability of T/R-capable surface coils augments efficiency significantly and encourages higher resolution scanning techniques. The higher SNR of 3T also facilitates the use of smaller fields of view, thinner slices, and larger imaging matrices. The greater susceptibility sensitivity of 3T should make tissue mineralization easier to appreciate (Fig. 31). Instrumented joints can be imaged with

manageable artifact with high bandwidth, long ET FSE, and T1-weighted IR FSE techniques.

Clinical practice impact

Fundamentally, 3T offers twice the signal of 1.5T. The overall power of 3T easily allows creation of studies that are recognizably better—with higher resolution and greater patient-to-patient consistency—in the same or less time than those that are practical at 1.5T.

For neurologic applications, 3T images are higher in resolution than are those at 1.5T, while maintaining higher SNR. Scan times are similar to or shorter than those at 1.5T, depending on the type of scan and goals of the imager. SNR and resolution contribute to better lesion definition and delineation (Fig. 32).

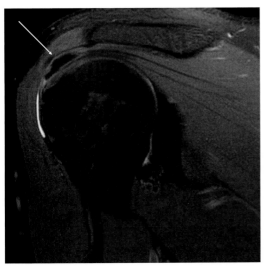

Figure 31 Fat suppressed FSE study reveals hydroxyapatite deposition.

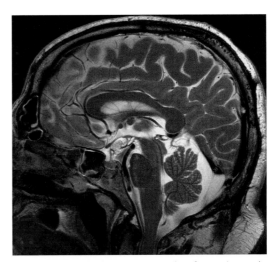

Figure 32 1024 × 384, 3-mm study of a patient who has a suprasellar lipoma. Note the z-axis uniformity of signal from convexity through foramen magnum on this study obtained with an 8-channel head coil.

The demands of small-part orthopedic work can exceed the capability of 1.5T to deliver in clinically feasible scan times. The combination of the inherent signal boost of 3T and dedicated surface coils produce a vast improvement in delineation of small structures, such as the triangular fibrocartilage complex and the intrinsic ligaments of the wrist (see Fig. 29). The greater image quality that 3T generates is met with enthusiasm from orthopedic referrers.

The ability of 3T to deliver thinner slices at higher in-plane resolution in body-imaging applications also has led to increased clinician preference for 3T. Near isotropic resolution acquisitions that are obtained at transient physiologic phases (eg, early-late arterial) allow diagnostic quality multiplanar reformatting. Hepatic and delayed-phase images at the same slice thickness and nearly the same in-plane spatial resolution of multichannel CT has facilitated abdominal and pelvic lesion detection and characterization significantly. More accurate and definitive interpretations have encouraged a shift toward 3T—as well as to MR imaging—from other methods of lesion assessment (Fig. 33).

At 1.5T, traditional MRA techniques suffer from lower spatial resolution and a lack of physiologic information, when compared with gold standard conventional angiography. The combination of an eight-channel surface coil at 3T and novel time-resolved acquisition techniques has overcome both of these hurdles. MR imaging now routinely delivers what only a catheter study could before—high spatial resolution, multiphase vascular assessment during the full cycle of vascular transit with complete freedom from interference from venous overlay. The surgeon's response to these superior, physiologic studies has been impressive, and has been a big factor in reducing the number of conventional angiographic studies that we are asked to perform.

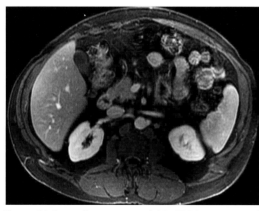

Figure 33 3-mm fat suppressed 3D GRE image reveals a spiculated pancreatic head mass consistent with carcinoma.

Summary

3T MRI is ready to meet the needs of clinical practice. SAR limitations are minimized by technical advances and surface coils are available for all core applications. With appropriate adjustments to scanning protocols, one can master the challenges of scanning at 3T; studies of the brain, spine, chest, abdomen, pelvis, vasculature, and extremities can be consistently higher in quality than are those obtained at 1.5T.

The superior studies that are obtainable at 3T have great appeal to clinicians who are sophisticated about MR technology in areas, such as neurology, orthopedics, vascular surgery, and oncology, and encourage a shift in referrals toward practices that invest in higher field technology. The greater sensitivity to magnetic susceptibility offers unique benefits in functional neuroimaging, and available software/hardware packages enhance clinical setting feasibility, which adds a source of new referrals. The greater overall signal of 3T can be manipulated to make scanning more comfortable and with less motion artifact because scan times could be half as long. Spectacular anatomic delineation that is provided by high-definition scanning at true 1024 resolution can improve preoperative assessment and may improve sensitivity to smaller lesions.

3T provides practices with an advantage that is sought increasingly by high field strength purchasers in a competitive market. Only cost considerations stand in the way of the eventual domination of 3T systems in the high field strength market.

References

[1] Tanenbaum LN. 3.0 T MRI in clinical practice. Appl Radiol 2005;34(1):8–17.

[2] Tanenbaum LN. 3.0 T MRI: ready for clinical practice [letter]. AJNR Am J Neuroradiol 2004; 25:1626–7.

[3] International Electrotechnical Commission. Medical electrical equipment – part 2: particular requirements for the safety of magnetic resonance equipment for medical diagnosis. International Electrotechnical Commission; 2002.

[4] Pruessmann KP. Parallel imaging at high field strength: synergies and joint potential. Top Magn Reson Imag 2004;15(4):237–44.

[5] Foster JR, Hall DA, Summerfield AQ, et al. Sound-level measurements and calculations of safe noise dosage during EPI at 3.0 T. J Magn Reson Imaging 2000;12:157–63.

[6] von Falkenhausen M, Gieseke1 J, Morakkabati-Spitz N, et al. Liver MRI at 3.0 T. Feasibility and limitations. Fortschr Geb Rontgenstr 2004;176.

[7] Frayne R, Goodyear B, Dickhoff P, et al. Magnetic resonance imaging at 3.0 T: challenges and

advantages in clinical neurological imaging. Invest Radiol 2003;38(7):385–402.

[8] Stollberger R, Fazekas F. Improved perfusion and tracer kinetic imaging using parallel imaging. Top Magn Reson Imag 2004;15(4):245–55.

[9] Field AS, Alexander AL. Diffusion tensor imaging in cerebral tumor diagnosis and therapy. Top Magn Reson Imag 2004;15(5):315–24.

[10] Roberts T, Rowley H. Diffusion weighted magnetic resonance imaging in stroke. Eur J Radiol 2003;45(3):185–94.

[11] Kruger G, Kastup A, Glover GH. Neuroimaging at 1.5T and 3.0 T: comparison of oxygenation-sensitive magnetic resonance imaging. Magn Reson Med 2001;45:595–604.

[12] Campeau NG, Huston J, Bernstein MA, et al. Magnetic resonance angiography at 3.0 T: initial clinical experience. Top Magn Reson Imag 2001; 12(3):183–204.

[13] Bernstein MA, Huston III J, Lin C, Gibbs GF, Felmlee JP. High-resolution intracranial and cervical MRA at 3.0 T: technical considerations and initial experience. Magn Reson Med 2001; 46(5):955–62.

[14] Larsson EM, Stahlberg F. 3.0 Tesla magnetic resonance imaging of the brain. Better morphological and functional images with higher magnetic field strength. Lakartidningen 2005; 102(7):460–3.

[15] Schmitt F, Grosu D, Mohr C, et al. 3.0 Tesla MRI: successful results with higher field strengths. Radiologe 2004;44(1):31–47.

[16] Leiner T, de Vries M, Hoogeveen R, et al. Contrast-enhanced peripheral MR angiography at 3.0 Tesla: initial experience with a whole-body scanner in healthy volunteers. J Magn Reson Imaging 2003; 17:609–14.

[17] Peterson D, Duensing GR, Caserta J, et al. An MR transceive phased array designed for spinal cord imaging at 3 Tesla: preliminary investigations of spinal cord imaging at 3T. Invest Radiol 2003; 38(7):428–35.

ELSEVIER SAUNDERS

MAGNETIC
RESONANCE
IMAGING CLINICS

Magn Reson Imaging Clin N Am (2006) 17–26

Abdominal MR Imaging at 3T

Elmar M. Merkle MD[a],*, Brian M. Dale PhD[b], Erik K. Paulson MD[a]

- The physics of abdominal 3T MR imaging
  Gain in signal-to-noise ratio at 3T
  Chemical shift artifacts
  Susceptibility artifacts
  Standing wave and conductivity artifacts
- Modifications of MR sequences to address
  specific ultrahigh-field issues
  Coronal turbo spin echo T2-weighted half Fourier single shot turbo spin echo sequence
  Axial gradient echo T1-weighted in- and opposed-phase sequence
- Summary
- References

Over the past 2 years, ultrahigh-field whole-body 3T magnetic resonance (MR) systems have been installed in numerous institutions worldwide, and are being used increasingly clinically. Besides market considerations, the main reason to purchase an ultrahigh-field MR system is the anticipated two-fold improvement in signal-to-noise ratio (SNR) compared with a standard 1.5T MR scanner. This gain in SNR can be kept and used directly to improve the quality of SNR-limited applications, or it can be traded for improved temporal or spatial resolution using parallel acquisition techniques. Although the number of accessory receiving coils had been limited in the past, the spectrum of receiver coils that is offered by the vendors has increased significantly over the past 12 months; multichannel torso array receive-only coils are now available on all whole-body 3T MR systems (Fig. 1). The increased availability of accessory coils should lead to increased clinical use of 3T units.

For various indications in the brain and musculoskeletal system, ultrahigh-field MR imaging has demonstrated certain advantages compared with standard high-field imaging; however, only a few scientific studies have been published that described the use of 3T MR systems in the chest, abdomen, and pelvis [1–10]. Insights gained in musculoskeletal or neuroimaging research at 3T cannot be transferred to body MR imaging, because MR sequence protocols, tissue properties, motion effects, certain artifacts, and object size differ significantly in abdominal imaging. It is not clear which patient groups will benefit from an ultrahigh-field abdominal MR study, and which patient groups should remain on a 1.5T MR scanner.

This article illustrates the underlying physical principles of abdominal MR imaging at 3T, and their impact on SNR, susceptibility artifacts, chemical shift artifacts, and standing-wave effects. Abdominal MR sequence protocols also are discussed with emphasis on the sequence modifications that are required during ultrahigh-field MR imaging. Finally, basic recommendations are provided to help identify patient groups that are likely to benefit from an ultrahigh-field MR study and patient groups that probably should undergo a standard 1.5T abdominal MR examination.

[a] Department of Radiology, Duke University Medical Center, Erwin Road, Duke North, Durham, NC 27710, USA
[b] Siemens Medical Solutions, Cary, NC, USA
*Corresponding author.
E-mail address: elmar.merkle@duke.edu (E.M. Merkle).

doi:10.1016/j.mric.2005.12.001

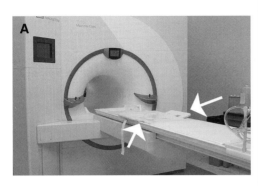
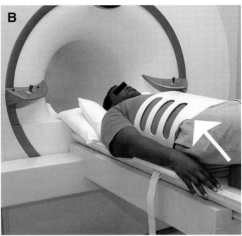
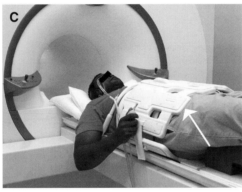

Figure 1 Magnetom TRIO (Siemens Medical Solutions), an ultrahigh-field whole body MR system with a dedicated receive only eight-channel torso array coil (USA Instruments, Aurora, Ohio). (*A*) The posterior four elements (*arrows*) of the dedicated receive only eight-channel torso array coil. (*B*) Usually, the patient is positioned "head first, supine" for abdominal MR examinations. Note the additional distance holder or "spacer" (*arrow*), which prevents the anterior and posterior receiver coil elements from overlapping laterally in slim patients. (*C*) The anterior four elements (*arrow*) of the dedicated receive only eight-channel torso array coil. (Courtesy of Siemens Medical Solutions, Cary, NC; with permission.)

The physics of abdominal 3T MR imaging

Gain in signal-to-noise ratio at 3T

The idea that twice the magnetic field will give twice the SNR is appealing, and at first it seems correct because the energy difference between the relaxed and unrelaxed states is approximately proportional to the main magnetic field strength (B_0) as seen below. Equations 1 and 2 are the result of developing this idea to obtain an expression for the SNR in MR imaging [11].

$$SNR_{SE} \propto B_0 V \sqrt{\frac{N_{PE}N_{PA}N_{AV}}{BW}} \left(1 - e^{-TR/T1}\right) e^{-TE/T2}$$

(1)

(SNR_{SE}, SNR for a spin echo pulse sequence; V, voxel volume; N_{PE}, number of acquired phase encode lines; N_{PA}, number of acquired partitions; N_{AV}, number of signals averaged; BW, receiver bandwidth per pixel; TR, repetition time; T1, longitudinal relaxation time; TE, echo time; T2, transverse relaxation time)

$$SNR_{GRE} \propto B_0 V \sqrt{\frac{N_{PE}N_{PA}N_{AV}}{BW}}$$
$$\frac{\sin(\theta)\left(1 - e^{-TR/T1}\right)}{\left(1 - e^{-TR/T1}\cos(\theta)\right)} e^{-TE/T2}$$

(2)

(SNR_{GRE}, SNR for a spoiled gradient echo sequence; Θ, flip angle)

Note that in equations 1 and 2, the term under the square root is the total time spent sampling the MR signal. Therefore, SNR is proportional to B_0, V, the square root of the total sampling time, and some sequence-specific contrast-related terms. Specific absorption rate (SAR) limitations can affect the SNR in a complicated manner by impacting other sequence specific parameters (eg, TR, FA).

It is well known that T1 increases at higher magnetic field strengths, which causes a decrease in SNR (see equations 1 and 2) [1,12]. Conversely, T2 seems to be independent of the B_0 [12], although one recently published study by de Bazelaire and colleagues [1] suggested a marked decrease of T2 for various abdominal tissues at higher magnetic field strengths. If the data of de Bazelaire and colleagues represent a general trend, then the T2 effect would reduce further the gain in SNR for long TE protocols at ultrahigh field. Equations 1 and 2 can be used in either case to determine the theoretic maximum relative gain in SNR during liver MR. The following calculations use the optimistic assumption that T2 is independent of B_0; however, by assuming only an increase in T1 and ignoring any potential decrease in the T2 relaxation time, the calculated SNR improvements may be too high. For turbo spin echo (TSE)-based T2-weighted sequences, such as half Fourier single shot turbo spin echo (HASTE), an approximately 1.8-fold increase in SNR can be obtained if critical MR sequence parameters, such as the TE, TR, BW, and flip angle (FA)/refocusing angle, are kept constant. For gradient echo–based T1-weighted sequences, such as fast low-angle shot (FLASH) or volume-interpolated breath-hold examination (VIBE), a 1.6- to 1.7-fold increase in SNR can be obtained (if sequence parameters are identical). Thus, the theoretic twofold increase in SNR at 3T, compared with 1.5T MR imaging, generally will not be obtained without sequence parameter optimization. Table 1 provides

a more detailed overview of the theoretic gain in SNR at 3T in various abdominal organs.

A second major factor with a negative impact on the gain in SNR is related to SAR, a measure of energy deposition within the human body. When all other parameters remain constant, SAR is proportional to the square of the field strength, so by doubling B_0, the SAR increases by a factor of four. Therefore, body MR imaging at 3T almost always runs at the upper limits of the allowed SAR deposition. To maintain a SAR that is less than the allowable limits, protocol adjustments (eg, increase of the TR, decrease in the number of slices, decrease of the FA) frequently are necessary. These adjustments are undesirable because they increase scan time, reduce anatomic coverage, alter contrast, or further reduce the gain in SNR at 3T.

Finally, much of the radiofrequency (RF) transmitter and receiver technology at 1.5T is mature compared with the newer technology at 3T.

Chemical shift artifacts

The chemical shift artifact of the first kind is due to a difference in the resonant frequency between water and fat, and is seen only along the frequency-encoding axis and the slice-selection dimension [13] (the axes where gradients are applied during RF reception or transmission, respectively). This difference in resonant frequency is directly proportional to B_0, and has been measured to be approximately 3.5 ppm, which results in a difference of about 225 Hz at 1.5T, or a difference of about 450 Hz at 3T. This difference causes a chemical shift misregistration wherever fat spins in one location precess at the same frequency as water spins in another location. In body imaging it is seen most easily around the kidneys. The chemical shift artifact of the first kind appears as a hypointense band, one to several pixels in width, toward the lower part of the readout gradient field, and as a hyperintense band toward the higher part of the readout gradient field. At a constant in-plane resolution and receiver bandwidth, the chemical shift artifact of the first kind will be twice as wide at 3T compared with 1.5T. Usually, this enhanced chemical shift artifact does not cause interpretive difficulties in clinical body MR imaging at ultrahigh field; however, it may be problematic in selected scenarios, such as the search for a subcapsular renal hematoma or an intramural aortic hematoma. In these cases, the receiver bandwidth can be increased to reduce the chemical shift artifact of the first kind. Unfortunately, this comes at the expense of SNR—doubling the receiver bandwidth will decrease the SNR gain by approximately 30% (see equations 1 and 2). Another option is to repeat the MR pulse sequence with a chemical shift fat saturation,

Table 1: Theoretic change in signal-to-noise ratio in various abdominal organs at 3T compared with 1.5T

	Liver	Kidney	Spleen
T1 and T2 relaxation times (ms)[a]			
T1 time (1.5T)	493	652	782
T1 time (3T)	641	774	984
T2 time (for 1.5T and 3T)	43	58	62
SNR change at 3T compared with 1.5T			
HASTE identical sequence parameters	1.82	1.85	1.77
FLASH identical sequence parameters	1.70	1.78	1.69
VIBE identical sequence parameters	1.61	1.73	1.63
HASTE actual sequence parameters	5.55	4.32	3.93
FLASH actual sequence parameters	1.06	1.06	0.97
VIBE actual sequence parameters	0.97	0.80	0.85

[a] *Data from* Bottomley PA, Foster TH, Argersinger RE, et al. A review of normal tissue hydrogen NMR relaxation times and relaxation mechanisms from 1–100 MHz: dependence on tissue type, NMR frequency, temperature, species, excision, and age. Med Phys 1984;11(4):425–48.

inversion nulling, or water excitation, which will eliminate chemical shift artifacts, allow imaging at the lower bandwidth, and return the 30% loss in SNR.

The chemical shift artifact of the second kind is based on an intravoxel phase-cancellation effect where fat and water exist in the same voxel. It is not limited to the frequency-encoding axis, but may be seen in all voxels along a fat–water interface [13]. The size of this artifact does not increase with B_0; however, the TE for obtaining this artifact needs to be adjusted at ultrahigh field because the frequency difference is twice as large compared with standard 1.5T MR systems (as described in the section on chemical shift artifact of the first kind). At 3T, fat and water protons are in-phase at TEs of 2.2 ms, 4.4 milliseconds, 6.6 milliseconds, and so on, and out-of-phase (also referred to as opposed phase) at 1.1 milliseconds, 3.3 milliseconds, 5.5 milliseconds, and so on. Although most vendors agree that both echoes (in-phase as well as opposed-phase echo) should be acquired during the same breath-hold to avoid misregistration, there is no consensus on which pair of echoes to acquire. Currently, acquiring the first opposed-phase echo at an ultrashort TE of 1.1 milliseconds and the first in-phase echo only 1.1 milliseconds later at 2.2 milliseconds within the same breath-hold (analogous to the echo collection on a 1.5T MR system with TEs of 2.2 milliseconds for opposed-phase and 4.4 milliseconds for in-phase imaging) requires unacceptably high receiver bandwidths. Thus, the second or third in-phase or opposed-phase echo needs to be collected. Currently, the in-phase MR signal is collected at a TE of 2.5 milliseconds (first in-phase signal) on ultrahigh-field MR systems that are manufactured by General Electric Health Care (Waukesha, Wisconsin) and the opposed-phase signal is collected at 5.8 milliseconds (third opposed-phase signal). Conversely, on 3T MR systems that are manufactured by Siemens Medical Solutions (Erlangen, Germany), the opposed-phase MR signal typically is collected at a TE of 1.5 milliseconds (first opposed-phase signal) and the in-phase signal is collected at 4.9 milliseconds (second in-phase signal). Although this discrepancy in echo collection schemes between the vendors does not cause significant problems in the detection of microscopic fatty components, it does affect the visualization of T2* effects and susceptibility artifacts. In- and opposed-phase imaging allows pathologic conditions that involve accumulations of iron (eg, siderotic nodules, hemochromatosis, hemosiderosis) to be detected easily and characterized with a high degree of confidence. In cases of iron storage disease, the hepatic parenchymal signal intensity decreases on the image with the longer TE because

of the continued T2* decay of the transverse magnetization. Thus, the liver parenchyma appear darker in the opposed-phase image from ultrahigh-field MR systems that are manufactured by General Electric Health Care and in the in-phase image from systems that are manufactured by Siemens Medical Solutions (Fig. 2).

The increased difference in resonant frequency between water and fat at 3T also is advantageous in many instances because it allows for a better separation of the fat and water peaks during MR spectroscopy, and for a better or faster fat suppression using other chemical shift techniques as well (eg, fat saturation and water excitation).

Susceptibility artifacts

Magnetic susceptibility is the extent to which a material becomes magnetized when placed within a magnetic field. Susceptibility artifacts occur as

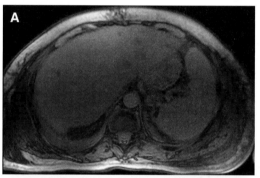

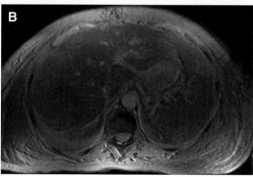

Figure 2 Visualization of T2* effects and susceptibility artifacts that are due to the double-echo approach during opposed-phase and in-phase MR imaging, using an ultrahigh-field 3T MR system, in a patient who had transfusional hemosiderosis. (*A*) Opposed-phase image acquired at a TE of 1.5 milliseconds shows liver and spleen signal intensity similar to muscle signal intensity. (*B*) In-phase image acquired at a TE of 4.9 milliseconds shows a marked decrease in signal intensity in the liver (from 114 to 70) and spleen (compare with *A*). Iron storage causes a significant local distortion of the nearby magnetic field which results in a significant shortening of the T2* relaxation time.

the result of static microscopic gradients or variations in the magnetic field strength that occur near the interfaces of materials of different magnetic susceptibility. Because the susceptibility of metal is much higher than that of soft tissue, these artifacts usually are caused by metallic objects from previous surgical/interventional procedures near or in the imaging field of view (FOV). Susceptibility artifacts increase with the B_0, and are approximately twice as large, in terms of volume, at 3T compared with 1.5T [14]. This may be advantageous in selected cases because metal-related susceptibility artifacts from surgical clips or surgical debris may be seen better; however, it is possible that the enlarged susceptibility artifacts may obscure important findings at 3T MR imaging that may have been visualized at 1.5T. Metal-containing devices that are considered to be MR safe at 1.5T are not necessarily safe at 3T. All such metal-containing devices need to be rigorously tested at 3T before affected patients may undergo an MR examination at this field strength [15–20].

Susceptibility artifacts also occur next to gas-filled structures, such as the gas-filled bowel, because the susceptibility of gas is almost zero. Thus, bowel wall imaging in patients who have inflammatory bowel disease or patients who are referred for MR colonography may be more challenging at 3T; however, the enlarged susceptibility artifacts that are due to a gas–soft tissue interface also may be helpful in detecting gas (eg, intrahepatic pneumobilia or free intraperitoneal gas).

Standing wave and conductivity artifacts

In addition to the exacerbation of artifacts that are seen at 1.5T, some new artifacts begin to appear at 3T in body imaging. These artifacts are related to the higher frequency B_1 transmit fields that are used at ultrahigh field. The wavelength of the RF field at 128 MHz (Larmor frequency at 3T) is 234 cm in free space, which is much larger than the FOV for clinical body imaging; however, water and most body tissues have a high dielectric constant, which reduces the speed and wavelength of the RF field. This effect reduces the RF field wavelength from 234 cm in free space to about 30 cm in most human tissues (ie, water containing) [21]. This is on the order of the size of the FOV for many body applications, and can result in "standing wave" effects (often incorrectly called "dielectric resonance" effects [22]). As a result, strong signal variations across an image can be seen, especially brightening in regions away from the receiver coil or dark "holes" that are caused by constructive or destructive interference from the standing waves. These artifacts tend to become more pronounced the larger the region of interest is relative to the

wavelength (ie, in body imaging they are seen more in obese patients with a distended abdomen than in thin patients).

A rapidly changing magnetic field, like the RF field, induces a circulating electric field. When this happens in a conductive medium, such as most body tissues, a circulating electric current is established. This current acts like an electromagnet that opposes the changing magnetic field, and reduces the amplitude and dissipates the energy of the RF field. The more conductive the medium, the stronger the opposing electromagnet, and therefore, the greater the attenuation of the RF field. Thus, large amounts of highly conductive tissues can cause shielding effects that result in hypointense areas in the image where the RF field is attenuated partially [22].

These two effects can combine to cause particularly strong artifacts for 3T body MR imaging in pregnant women and patients who have ascites (Fig. 3). In these cases, the standing wave effects are more pronounced because of the enlarged abdomen relative to the RF wavelength, and there is greater RF field attenuation because of the increased amounts of highly conductive amniotic or ascitic fluid.

Recently, two vendors (Siemens Medical Solutions and General Electric Heath Care) introduced "RF cushions" to improve the homogeneity of the image during ultrahigh-field abdominal MR

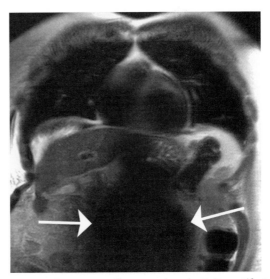

Figure 3 Severe standing-wave/conductivity artifact during ultrahigh-field MR imaging at 3T. Coronal HASTE image shows a marked signal loss in the center of the image (*arrows*) in a patient who had liver cirrhosis and ascites. Fluid accumulations within the peritoneal cavity enlarge the abdomen and increase the electrical conductivity within the FOV, which causes severe artifacts.

imaging (Fig. 4). These RF cushions may be used in conjunction with the body coil, as well as a dedicated receive-only torso array coil, and consist of a gel encapsulated in synthetic material. The gel is ultrasound gel, which has a high dielectric constant, is mixed with a highly concentrated gadolinium- or manganese-based MR contrast agent to eliminate the MR signal from the gel itself.

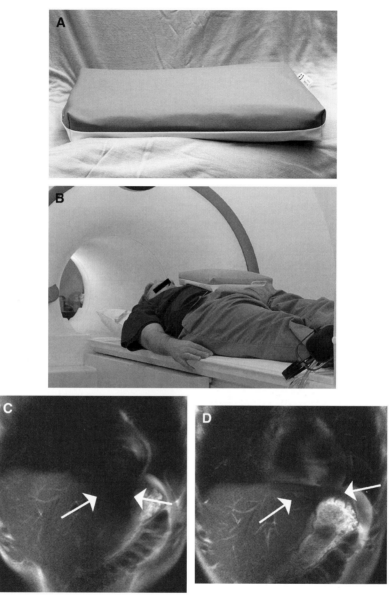

Figure 4 RF cushion to improve the homogeneity of the signal on T2-weighted sequences during ultrahigh-field abdominal MR imaging. (*A*) An RF cushion (Siemens Medical Solutions), which measures 36 cm × 26 cm × 3 cm [L × W × H]. The gray part is a simple foam pad, and the white part consists of a water-based gel mixed with a highly concentrated gadolinium-based MR contrast agent encapsulated in synthetic material. (*B*) Positioning of the RF cushion. If optimal RF homogeneity is desired, the RF cushion is positioned with the white side on the patient; however, this will result in a local B_0 field distortion that causes potential suboptimal fat saturation in this area. To obtain optimized RF homogeneity with improved fat saturation in the area of the anterior abdominal wall, the RF cushion is positioned with the gray side ("with distance") on the patient. (*C*) Coronal HASTE image acquired in a healthy male volunteer without the use of an RF cushion shows a marked signal loss (*arrows*) in the center of the image, which prevents evaluation of the left liver lobe. (*D*) After placement of an RF cushion, the quality of the coronal HASTE image is improved markedly (compare with *C*), and the left liver lobe is depicted adequately.

Modifications of MR sequences to address specific ultrahigh-field issues

An abdominal MR sequence protocol routinely consists of coronal single-shot TSE T2-weighted images (eg, HASTE), axial gradient echo in- and opposed-phase T1-weighted images, axial TSE T2-weighted images with fat saturation, and dynamic gradient echo T1-weighted images (eg, FLASH or VIBE) with fat saturation before and after the intravenous administration of gadolinium-based contrast agents (Figs. 5 and 6). These sequences represent the backbone of each abdominal breath-hold MR scan protocol, and are adjusted to meet the clinical indication for the MR examination and the specific needs of the patient (eg, the patient's breath-holding capabilities). Occasionally, these standard sequences are complemented by additional specialized MR sequences, such as the flow sensitive true-FISP (balanced fast imaging with steady state precession) to assess vascular problems or rapid acquisition with relaxation enhancement (RARE) as part of an MR cholangiography scan protocol (Fig. 7).

In general, MR sequence protocols that are established at 1.5T can be transferred to ultrahigh-field MR scanners; however, without modification, the outcome will be suboptimal and often—because of SAR limitations—the MR system does not execute the specific sequence without modification. Therefore, MR sequences have been and should continue to be optimized to meet the specific needs of ultra-high field MR imaging. In the following, these modifications are presented (eg, for TSE-based T2-weighted sequences and gradient echo–based T1-weighted sequences).

Coronal turbo spin echo T2-weighted half Fourier single shot turbo spin echo sequence

1.5T: TR/TE/FA/BW = 1010 milliseconds/126 milliseconds/180°/488 Hz/pixel

3T: TR/TE/FA/BW = 1000 milliseconds/82 milliseconds/136°/558 Hz/pixel

SAR limitations usually require a significant reduction of the 180°-refocusing pulses, which translates into a smaller gain in SNR and an alteration of image contrast. The SNR reduction is exacerbated by the higher receiver bandwidth at ultrahigh-field MR imaging. By decreasing the TE to 82 milliseconds, the gain in SNR is restored, but at the expense of some T2 contrast.

Overall, the coronal HASTE sequence that is used at 3T provides excellent image quality in normal-sized patients. Conductivity and standing wave artifacts can be severe in large patients who have ascites, but also can occur to a minor degree in thin patients (see Fig. 3). The same holds true for other T2-weighted TSE-based sequences, such as RARE, or recently introduced respiratory-triggered three-dimensional sequences that are used for MR cholangiography applications.

Hyperechoes are an appealing concept to solve the problem of SAR-related refocusing pulse reductions at ultrahigh-field TSE T2-weighted MR imaging, especially considering that SAR is proportional to the square of the FA if all other factors are held constant. This concept was described first by Hennig and colleagues [23,24], and is a novel spin-echo–based refocusing strategy by which the full coherence of magnetization that is submitted to a sequence of arbitrary RF pulses can be reinstalled. Hennig and colleagues developed an algorithm (based on the extended-phase graph algorithm) for calculation of the FAs that are required in a multiecho experiment to

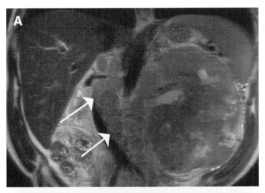

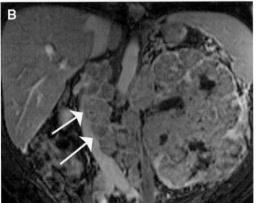

Figure 5 (*A*) Ultrahigh-field coronal HASTE image shows a left-sided renal cell cancer with extensive lymph node metastases (*arrows*) along the abdominal aorta and inferior vena cava. (*B*) Ultrahigh-field coronal VIBE image after gadolinium administration shows the primary renal tumor and the lymph node metastases (*arrows*). Note the homogeneous fat saturation.

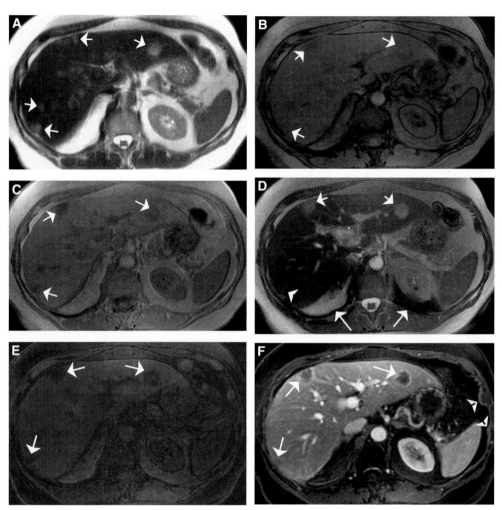

Figure 6 Ultrahigh-field MR examination in a patient who had ovarian cancer and subsequent peritoneal and hepatic metastases. (*A*) Axial HASTE image shows several hyperintense masses (*arrows*) within both lobes of the liver. (*B*) Axial opposed-phase image shows several hepatic masses (*arrows*) that appear predominantly hypointense. Note the chemical shift artifact of the second kind (aka India ink artifact) that appears similar to the one seen on 1.5T opposed-phase imaging. (*C*) Axial in-phase image shows hepatic masses (*arrows*) that appear hypointense. Note the chemical shift artifact of the first kind, which appears larger than the one usually seen on 1.5T in-phase imaging. The lower part of the readout gradient field is located on the left side in this case. (*D*) Axial TRUE-FISP image shows the hepatic masses (*short arrows*) are predominantly hyperintense. This specific sequence is sensitive to magnetic field inhomogeneity and results in bizarre signal alterations (eg, incomplete fat saturation [*arrows*]). In addition, focal lesions can be obscured as seen in the right hepatic lobe (*arrowhead*). (*E*) Axial VIBE shows hepatic masses as hypointense lesions (*arrows*). Note good fat saturation. (*F*) Axial VIBE after gadolinium administration shows hepatic metastases as hypointense lesions with rim enhancement (*arrows*). Note peritoneal implants (*arrowheads*).

generate echoes with predefined amplitudes. This algorithm can be used to optimize the echo envelope, and thus, the point spread function, while minimizing the total RF power deposition. Implementations at 3T, using echo trains with Gaussian and Lorentzian point spread functions, demonstrate a reduction in RF power by a factor of three to five while maintaining high image quality.

Axial gradient echo T1-weighted in- and opposed-phase sequence

- 1.5T: $TR/TE_1/TE_2/FA/BW$ = 100 milliseconds/ 2.38 milliseconds/5.07 milliseconds/70°/380 Hz/pixel
- 3T: $TR/TE_1/TE_2/FA/BW_1/BW_2$ = 216 milliseconds/1.52 milliseconds/4.90 milliseconds/ 71°/890 Hz/pixel/210 Hz/pixel

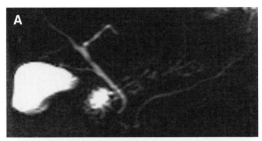

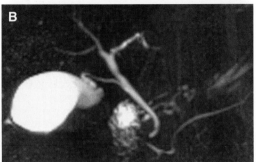

Figure 7 Ultrahigh-field MR cholangiopancreatography without pathologic findings. (*A*) Coronal RARE sequence shows normal depiction of the pancreatic and biliary ductal system. (*B*) Coronal three-dimensional T2-weighted TSE sequence, with respiratory triggering using a navigator technique, shows the same findings with significantly higher spatial resolution and higher SNR.

The most obvious changes in the sequence protocol are the adjustments of the in-phase and opposed-phase TEs at ultrahigh-field MR imaging. The receiver bandwidth also has been adjusted which has an impact on the SNR and the size of the chemical shift artifact of the first kind. By increasing the TR, the T1 contrast is maintained and the SNR is restored at the expense of acquisition time. Overall, the axial gradient echo T1-weighted in- and opposed-phase sequence provides excellent image quality and works as robustly at 3T as it does at 1.5T. Specifically, the standing wave and conductivity effects are less noticeable on gradient echo images than on TSE images. The same holds true for the VIBE and FLASH sequence, which also provide excellent image quality that is comparable to the image quality that radiologists are used to from 1.5T MR systems.

Summary

Body MR imaging at 3T is in its infancy, and should improve substantially over the next several years. Radiologists need to be aware of several limitations that are based on the laws of physics:

Overall, the gain in SNR at 3T will be less than twofold (without protocol alteration)

compared with a standard 1.5T MR system because of the increase in T1 at ultrahigh field. Typically, the gain in SNR is greater in T2-weighted sequences than in T1-weighted sequences, because longer TRs allow for a more complete recovery of the longitudinal magnetization, and T2 is independent of B_0. Thus, for example, patients who are referred for an MR cholangiography may benefit from an ultrahigh-field MR examination.

Chemical shift artifacts of the first kind are twice as large in ultrahigh-field MR imaging compared with standard 1.5T MR imaging. Conversely, chemical shift artifacts of the second kind do not increase in size, although the timing is altered. The increased difference in resonant frequency between water and fat at 3T also is advantageous because it allows for a better separation of the fat and water peak during MR spectroscopy, and allows better or faster fat suppression using chemical shift techniques, such as fat saturation or water excitation.

Susceptibility artifacts are approximately twice as large by volume on 3T MR imaging. Although patients who are referred for a "colon" study may be challenging at ultrahigh field, the search for "gas" (eg, free air or pneumobilia) should be easier. Patients with metal implants should undergo an MR examination at 3T only if the metal-containing device specifically has been proved to be MR safe at this field strength.

Usually, standing wave and conductivity effects are not seen in body imaging at a field strength of 1.5T. At 3T, these artifacts are most pronounced in pregnant women in the second and third trimester, because of the large amount of conductive amniotic fluid and the increased size of the abdomen. Therefore, fetal MR imaging generally should not be performed at 3T because of these artifacts and the increased safety concerns. The same holds true for patients with a large amount of ascites, who also are not well suited for an ultrahigh-field MR examination.

Except as noted above, most patients can undergo an abdominal MR imaging study at 3T with a reasonable outcome in terms of image quality.

References

[1] de Bazelaire CM, Duhamel GD, Rofsky NM, et al. MR imaging relaxation times of abdominal and pelvic tissues measured in vivo at 3.0 T: preliminary results. Radiology 2004;230(3):652–9.

[2] Katz-Brull R, Rofsky NM, Lenkinski RE. Breath-hold abdominal and thoracic proton MR spectroscopy at 3T. Magn Reson Med 2003;50(3):461–7.

[3] Sosna J, Rofsky NM, Gaston SM, et al. Determinations of prostate volume at 3-Tesla using an external phased array coil: comparison to pathologic specimens. Acad Radiol 2003;10(8):846–53.

[4] Bloch BN, Rofsky NM, Baroni RH, et al. 3 Tesla magnetic resonance imaging of the prostate with combined pelvic phased-array and endorectal coils: initial experience. Acad Radiol 2004;11(8):863–7.

[5] Sosna J, Pedrosa I, Dewolf WC, et al. MR imaging of the prostate at 3 Tesla: comparison of an external phased-array coil to imaging with an endorectal coil at 1.5 Tesla. Acad Radiol 2004;11(8):857–62.

[6] Greenman RL, Shirosky JE, Mulkern RV, et al. Double inversion black-blood fast spin-echo imaging of the human heart: a comparison between 1.5T and 3.0T. J Magn Reson Imaging 2003;17(6):648–55.

[7] Sommer T, Hackenbroch M, Hofer U, et al. Coronary MR angiography at 3.0 T versus that at 1.5 T: initial results in patients suspected of having coronary artery disease. Radiology 2005;234(3):718–25.

[8] Michaely HJ, Nael K, Schoenberg SO, et al. The feasibility of spatial high-resolution magnetic resonance angiography (MRA) of the renal arteries at 3.0 T. Rofo 2005;177(6):800–4.

[9] Morakkabati-Spitz N, Gieseke J, Kuhl C, et al. 3.0-T high-field magnetic resonance imaging of the female pelvis: preliminary experiences. Eur Radiol 2005;15(4):639–44.

[10] Lutterbey G, Gieseke J, von Falkenhausen M, et al. Lung MRI at 3.0 T: a comparison of helical CT and high-field MRI in the detection of diffuse lung disease. Eur Radiol 2005;15(2):324–8.

[11] Edelstein WA, Glover GH, Hardy CJ, et al. The intrinsic signal-to-noise ratio in NMR imaging. Magn Reson Med 1986;3(4):604–18.

[12] Bottomley PA, Foster TH, Argersinger RE, et al. A review of normal tissue hydrogen NMR relaxation times and relaxation mechanisms from 1–100 MHz: dependence on tissue type, NMR frequency, temperature, species, excision, and age. Med Phys 1984;11(4):425–48.

[13] Elster AE, Burdette JHMR. Artifacts. In: Elster AE, Burdette JH, editors. Questions and answers in magnetic resonance imaging. 2nd edition. St. Louis (MO): Mosby; 2001. p. 123–47.

[14] Lewin JS, Duerk JL, Jain VR, et al. Needle localization in MR-guided biopsy and aspiration: effects of field strength, sequence design, and magnetic field orientation. AJR Am J Roentgenol 1996;166(6):1337–45.

[15] Sommer T, Maintz D, Schmiedel A, et al. High field MR imaging: magnetic field interactions of aneurysm clips, coronary artery stents and iliac artery stents with a 3.0 Tesla MR system. Rofo 2004;176(5):731–8.

[16] Shellock FG. Biomedical implants and devices: assessment of magnetic field interactions with a 3.0-Tesla MR system. J Magn Reson Imaging 2002;16(6):721–32.

[17] Shellock FG, Tkach JA, Ruggieri PM, et al. Cardiac pacemakers, ICDs, and loop recorder: evaluation of translational attraction using conventional ("long-bore") and "short-bore" 1.5- and 3.0-Tesla MR systems. J Cardiovasc Magn Reson 2003;5(2):387–97.

[18] Baker KB, Nyenhuis JA, Hrdlicka G, et al. Neurostimulation systems: assessment of magnetic field interactions associated with 1.5- and 3-Tesla MR systems. J Magn Reson Imaging 2005;21(1):72–7.

[19] Shellock FG, Gounis M, Wakhloo A. Detachable coil for cerebral aneurysms: in vitro evaluation of magnetic field interactions, heating, and artifacts at 3T. AJNR Am J Neuroradiol 2005;26(2):363–6.

[20] Shellock FG, Forder JR. Drug eluting coronary stent: in vitro evaluation of magnet resonance safety at 3 Tesla. J Cardiovasc Magn Reson 2005;7(2):415–9.

[21] Haacke EM, Brown RW, Thompson MR, et al. Magnetic resonance imaging - physical principles and sequence design. 1st edition. New York: John Wiley & Sons; 1999.

[22] Collins CM, Liu W, Schreiber W, et al. Central brightening due to constructive interference with, without, and despite dielectric resonance. J Magn Reson Imaging 2005;21(2):192–6.

[23] Hennig J, Scheffler K. Hyperechoes. Magn Reson Med 2001;46(1):6–12.

[24] Hennig J, Weigel M, Scheffler K. Calculation of flip angles for echo trains with predefined amplitudes with the extended phase graph (EPG)-algorithm: principles and applications to hyperecho and TRAPS sequences. Magn Reson Med 2004;51(1):68–80.

**ELSEVIER
SAUNDERS**

MAGNETIC
RESONANCE
IMAGING CLINICS

Magn Reson Imaging Clin N Am (2006) 27–40

3T MR Imaging of the Musculoskeletal System (Part I): Considerations, Coils, and Challenges

R. Richard Ramnath MD

- Increased signal-to-noise ratio at 3T
- Increased spatial resolution at 3T
- Decreased scan time at 3T
- Coil selection
  - *Knee coils*
  - *Shoulder coils*
  - *Wrist coils*
  - *Elbow coils*
  - *Ankle coils*
  - *Hip coils*
- Specific absorption rate

- Parallel imaging
- Susceptibility artifact
- Chemical shift artifact
- Pulsation artifact
- Truncation artifact
- Dielectric resonance (field focusing)
- T1 relaxation times
- T2 decay times
- Summary
- References

As clinical musculoskeletal MR imaging transitions from 1.5T systems to the now widely available 3T systems, the advantages of higher field strength in the evaluation of musculoskeletal disorders has become apparent. The improved signal-to-noise ratio (SNR) can be harnessed to improve imaging times and spatial resolution. The end result is better image quality and potentially increased diagnostic accuracy. Several challenges, however, have to be considered to realize the potential of 3T imaging. There are many issues that pertain specifically to the extremities and joints that require consideration, such as specific absorption rate (SAR), chemical shift artifact, susceptibility artifact, pulsation artifact, T1 time prolongation, and T2 time shortening.

In addition, the development of surface extremity coils that are designed to maximize 3T imaging capability has been slower than the advances in 3T MR systems. Despite that fact, many extremity coils from various manufacturers are available for the three major MR vendors that can harness much of the gain in magnetic field strength. The images that are produced from these coils are superb and certainly outperform those that are seen from 1.5T systems; however, the full potential of coil technology has yet to be realized, as development in the number of coil channels and parallel imaging capabilities slowly gains speed.

At the current state of 3T extremity coil availability, image quality already has surpassed most expectations, and the constant improvements in coil technology and imaging techniques bode well for an exciting future in 3T musculoskeletal imaging.

Increased signal-to-noise ratio at 3T

The clear advantage of 3T scanners is the improved SNR. An in-depth understanding of how the SNR is obtained is necessary to know the appropriate

Neuroskeletal Imaging, 1344 South Apollo Boulevard, Suite 406, Melbourne, FL 32901, USA
E-mail address: rramnath@neuroskeletal.com

doi:10.1016/j.mric.2006.01.001

application and limitations of such a signal. The signal that is gained at higher field strengths is related, predictably, to the equilibrium magnetization, voxel size, and resonance frequency as demonstrated in this equation [1–3]:

$S \alpha \omega_0 M_0 V = S \alpha \omega_0 M_0$ (for a given voxel size)

S = signal, ω_0 = resonance frequency, M_0 = equilibrium magnetization, V = voxel size

The Larmor equation describes the relationship of the resonance frequency and the main magnetic field as such:

$\omega_0 = \gamma B_0$

ω_0 = resonance frequency, γ = gyromagnetic ratio, B_0 = main magnetic field

The Larmor equation can be substituted into the first equation:

$S \alpha \gamma B_0 M_0$

If the equilibrium magnetization is proportional to B_0 by:

$M_0 \alpha \rho \gamma^2 h^2 B_0 / 4kT$

or

$M_0 \alpha B_0$

Then, by substitution:

$S \alpha \gamma B_0 B_0$ or $S \alpha B_0^2$

Therefore, the signal at 3T is four times the signal at 1.5T; however, the story does not end there. To arrive at an estimation of SNR, a consideration of noise is necessary. Because noise (N) is proportional to the resonance frequency (ω_0):

$N \alpha \omega_0$

And by substituting the Larmor equation:

$N \alpha \gamma B_0$

Therefore, the noise at 3T is two times the noise at 1.5T. This leaves us with an SNR of two (4S/2N) times the SNR at 1.5T.

Increased spatial resolution at 3T

With the improved SNR at 3T, one can immediately take advantage of increasing the spatial resolution in several fashions [1–3]. To understand how to accomplish this, a discussion of the relationship between SNR and spatial resolution is helpful. SNR is proportional to slice thickness and in-plane resolution as follows:

$SNR = K \cdot (VxVyVz) \cdot \sqrt{(NxNyNex/BW)}$

or

$SNR \alpha (FOVx/Nx) \cdot (FOVy/Ny) \cdot Vz \cdot \sqrt{(Nx \cdot Ny)}$

K = constant, Vx = voxel size in x direction, Vy = voxel size in y direction, Vz = voxel size in z direction, Nx = number of frequency encoding steps, Ny = number of phase encoding steps, Nex = number of excitations, BW = bandwidth, FOVx = field of view in the x direction, FOVy = field of view in the y direction

If the SNR at 1.5T is one half of the SNR at 3T, then the following equation applies:

$1/2(SNR_{3T}) \alpha 1/2((FOVx/Nx) \cdot (FOVy/Ny) \cdot Vz \cdot \sqrt{(Nx \cdot Ny)})$

Therefore, to keep a 3T scan at the same SNR as at 1.5T, one may decrease the slice thickness by half for two dimensions (2D), while maintaining in-plane resolution:

$SNR_{1.5\,T} \alpha 1/2Vz \cdot (FOVx/Nx) \cdot (FOVy/Ny) \cdot \sqrt{(Nx \cdot Ny)}$

Or one may choose to double the in-plane resolution in the x and y directions, while maintaining the slice thickness:

$SNR_{1.5\,T} \alpha Vz \cdot (FOVx/2Nx) \cdot (FOVy/2Ny) \cdot \sqrt{(2Nx \cdot Ny)}$

or

$SNR_{1.5\,T} \alpha Vz \cdot 1/2(FOVx/Nx) \cdot 1/2(FOVy/Ny) \cdot \sqrt{4NxNy}$

or

$SNR_{1.5\,T} \alpha Vz \cdot 1/4((FOVx/Nx) \cdot (FOVy/Ny)) \cdot 2\sqrt{NxNy}$

or

$SNR_{1.5\,T} \alpha 2/4((FOVx/Nx) \cdot (FOVy/Ny)) \cdot Vz \cdot \sqrt{(Nx \cdot Ny)}$

For example, if a 2D fast spin echo (FSE) coronal knee sequence is obtained with a 4-mm slice thickness and a 256 × 192 in-plane resolution at 1.5T, one may adjust the resolution as follows for a 3T scan (while maintaining a similar SNR as the 1.5T scan):

2-mm slice thickness and 256 × 192 in-plane resolution

or

4-mm slice thickness and 512 × 192 in-plane resolution

Any variation of these parameters also may be used effectively as long as the SNR equation is fulfilled. It is important to realize that doubling the slice direction resolution, while also doubling the in-plane resolution, would violate the equation and push the system beyond its capabilities.

Decreased scan time at 3T

The improved SNR at 3T may be exploited to improve spatial resolution, and to decrease scanning time [1–3] and increase patient throughput. This can be deduced from the following discussion. The SNR is proportional to the number of acquisitions (time) as follows:

$$SNR = K \cdot (VxVyVz) \cdot \sqrt{(NxNyNex/BW)}$$

or

$$SNR_{3T} \, \alpha \, \left(\sqrt{N_{ex}}\right)_{3T}$$

Therefore, if the SNR at 1.5T is one half of the SNR at 3T, then to maintain the SNR of 1.5T, one could decrease the number of acquisitions to one fourth:

$$1/2\left(SNR_{3T}\right) \, \alpha \, \sqrt{1/4}\left(N_{acq}\right)$$

Theoretically, one could decrease scan times to one fourth if the sequences obtained at 1.5T were 4 NEX (number of excitations) or four acquisitions. In that scenario, if the average knee examination at 1.5T is 20 minutes (not including positioning time and prescanning time), then the examination theoretically could be reduced to 5 minutes on 3T. Consequently, patient schedule time slots could be reduced from 30 minutes to 10 to 15 minutes. If an MR scanner operates from 7 AM to 11 PM (16-hour day), one could increase patient throughput from 32 patients per day to 64 or 96 patients per day.

Because not all sequences are obtained with 4 or higher NEX at 1.5T, the actual reduction in scan time is not quite one fourth. For instance, in the author's practice, if we decrease scan times for a knee MR imagining using a 1 NEX per sequence and a matrix of 256 × 192, the total scan time would be approximately 6:13 (Table 1). The image quality from this set of parameters rivals a 1.5T examination.

Additional time for patient positioning, technologist scan set-up, and radiofrequency (RF)

prescanning likely would bring this to a realistic scan slot of 15 minutes. Furthermore, adjustments in slice thickness, number of slices, in-plane resolution, repetition time (TR), and echo train length (ETL) would have effects on the actual time.

Another benefit of decreased scan times is improved patient tolerance and decreased motion artifact. This would have the added effect of eliminating the need to repeat sequences, and thereby, would reduce overall scan time further relative to a 1.5T scanner. In my musculoskeletal examinations, I have chosen a compromise between decreased scan times and increased spatial resolution, so that I could demonstrate improved image quality to our referring orthopedic surgeons, while satisfying the patients' need to decrease time spent in the magnet.

Coil selection

As rapidly as the manufacturers of MR imaging systems have improved and fine-tuned 3T MR systems, coil design and development have been unable to demonstrate the same rapid pace. A brief discussion of coil designs is needed to understand the latest in coil development and applications to 3T MR imaging. There are two major fundamental coil designs in regards to the RF pulses that are used in MR imaging: transmit-receive and receive-only. Transmit-receive coils have the ability to apply RF pulses into the body part that is being imaged and to receive the signal that is obtained after RF stimulation [4]. The classic transmit-receive coil is the body coil that is built into the MR imaging system; however, many surface or volume coils that were developed for the musculoskeletal system also take advantage of transmit-receive technology. Birdcage and saddle coils are the most common types of surface or volume coils with transmit-receive capability. Most available transmit-receive extremity coils use a quadrature coil element design, which obtains in-phase and out-of-phase signals to construct k-space [5]. Because they typically are transmit-receive, quadrature coil systems have the major advantage of reducing the SAR for an examination (see later discussion).

A unique and special type of coil design uses phased-array technology [6]. These coils use a series of highly specialized coil elements to obtain signal

Table 1: Reduction in scan time at 3T

COR FSE T2 FS	COR FSE T1	SAG FSE PD	SAG FSE T2 FS	AX FSE T2 FS	
ETL 12	ETL 3	ETL 6	ETL 12	ETL 12	Total
1:00	1:22	1:35	1:16	1:00	6:13

Scan times for each sequence in our knee exam using a 1 NEX per sequence and 256 × 192 matrix.
Abbreviations: AX, axial; COR, coronal; FS, fat saturation; SAG, sagittal.

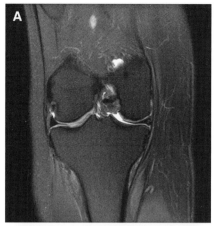

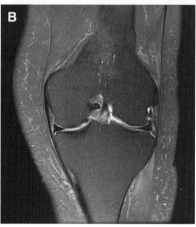

Figure 1 Coronal FSE T2-weighted sequences with fat saturation using two different 3T knee coils on two different patients. Similar imaging parameters were used in both sequences. (*A*) Medical Advances quadrature transmit-receive knee coil. (*B*) MRI Devices phased-array transmit-receive knee coil demonstrates improved SNR.

individually, and have the potential to provide spatial data for k-space construction. These coils improved the SNR compared with other coil designs and are necessary for the use of parallel imaging (see later discussion). Most phased-array coils are receive-only, which, on 3T systems, eliminates the SAR-friendly factor that is found in the conventional quadrature designs. Fig. 1 demonstrates the improvement in SNR that can be achieved by using a phased-array coil design.

The author's practice uses coils that are designed by three of the major coil manufacturers: USA Instruments (USA Instruments, Aurora, Ohio), Medical Advances (IGC-Medical Advances, Milwaukee, Wisconsin), and MRI Devices (MRI Devices, Gainesville, Florida). Although there are numerous coil manufacturers, the author's experience has been with these particular companies.

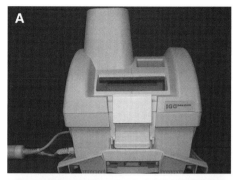

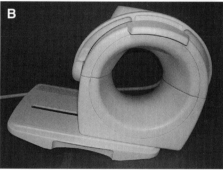

Figure 2 Two knee coils used with the author's 3T system. (*A*) Medical Advances quadrature design transmit-receive knee coil. (*B*) MRI Devices eight-channel phased-array transmit-receive knee coil.

Knee coils

USA Instruments and Medical Advances (Fig. 2A) have designed transmit-receive quadrature knee coils, which have the advantage of SAR reduction. The Medical Advances knee coil also incorporates a "chimney component," which allows the dual purpose of foot and ankle imaging with the foot in neutral position.

MRI Devices has developed an eight-channel, phased-array knee coil with parallel imaging capabilities (Fig. 2B). This coil has transmit-receive capability, which allows a potential reduction in SAR. In addition, the use of parallel imaging has SAR-saving features and can improve the versatility of the coil further. One drawback to this particular coil that is noted by many users is its smaller coil diameter, which can limit the ability to image large patients.

Several coil manufacturers are developing phased-array extremity coils with equal or more channels, and the next few months and years will see a dramatic increase in phased-array coil options at 3T.

Shoulder coils

The author's practice uses shoulder coils that are designed by two of the major coil manufacturers: USA

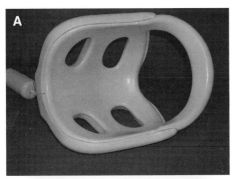

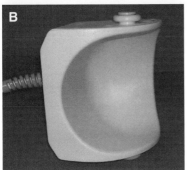

Figure 3 Two shoulder coils used with the author's 3T system. (*A*) USA Instruments three-channel receive-only phased-array coil. (*B*) MRI Devices eight-channel phased-array receive-only shoulder coil.

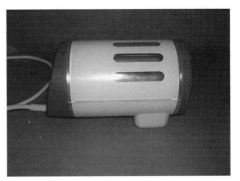

Figure 4 Mayo Clinic 3T wrist coil is a single-channel transmit-receive coil.

Instruments and MRI Devices (Fig. 3). USA Instruments and MRI Devices have designed phased-array, receive-only shoulder coils. In addition, the MRI Devices shoulder coil comes in large and small sizes to optimize patient positioning; it also comes in a quadrature design.

Whether due to distance from isocenter or coil design, our ability to harness the full potential of the increased 3T SNR with these coils has been suboptimal. Although we have seen an improvement in image quality compared with 1.5T scans, we are yet to achieve the spatial resolution for a given scan time as with other joints. The good news is that all the coil manufacturers are working feverishly to improve on shoulder coil design, including making phased-array, parallel-imaging compatible coil systems more easily accessible.

Wrist coils

Our practice uses a wrist coil that was designed by the Mayo Clinic (Rochester, Minnesota) (Fig. 4). This particular coil is a transmit-receive single-channel quadrature design. USA Instruments and MRI Devices have wrist coils for 3T. In addition, the MRI Devices wrist coil uses a phased-array design.

For optimal signal, the Mayo Clinic coil needs to be positioned as close to isocenter as possible. Therefore, all patients are positioned prone with

the arm above the head in the so-called "Superman" position. The author find that this coil provides robust signal and also uses it for finger imaging. The coil has a small diameter and cannot be used for elbow imaging in most patients. Furthermore, the field of view (FOV) is approximately 10 cm, and a large FOV wrist and hand image cannot be obtained.

A general purpose flex coil is available through GE systems (General Electric, Milwaukee, Wisconsin) for wrist imaging, if needed; however, the signal tends to be less impressive compared with the dedicated wrist coils (Fig. 5).

Elbow coils

The author's practice uses the quadrature transmit-receive Medical Advances knee coil (see Fig. 2A) or the transmit-receive eight-channel phased-array MRI Devices knee coil (see Fig. 2B) for elbow imaging, depending on the size of the patient.

For optimal signal, the coil is positioned as close to isocenter as possible. Therefore, all patients who are undergoing examination of their elbow, just like for the wrist, are positioned prone or on their side with the arm above the head in the so-called "Superman" position. The author prefers the MRI

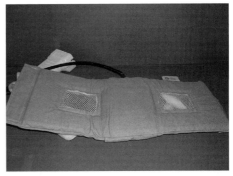

Figure 5 General purpose flex coil for multipurpose use can be used for wrist, elbow, or shoulder imaging.

Devices coil because of the excellent signal that is afforded by the phased-array design. Occasionally, larger patients need to be imaged in the wider diameter Medical Advances coil.

Ankle coils

The author's practice uses the Medical Advances transmit-receive quadrature knee coil with chimney component for foot and ankle imaging (see Fig. 2A). The chimney component allows for neutral ankle positioning. Typically, the signal that is obtained is rich, with only occasional problems with inhomogeneous fat saturation in the ankles and forefoot. The inhomogeneity often can be fixed by fastidiously positioning the coil closer to isocenter.

Hip coils

The USA Instruments torso eight-channel phased-array coil is extremely effective for hip and pelvis imaging (Fig. 6). There is excellent SNR for labral and cartilage detail. Furthermore, the parallel imaging capability allows for shortened scan times without a perceptible depreciation in signal.

Specific absorption rate

SAR is the term that is used to describe the energy that is deposited in a patient per unit of mass or weight. SAR increases with the strength of the magnetic field (see later discussion), which is a potential limitation in the clinical applicability of high-field strength systems. The U.S. Food and Drug Administration and the International Electrotechnical Committee set SAR safety limits of an increase in core body temperature of no more than 1°C. To operate within this limit, several specific power limits have been precalculated to minimize the degree of patient heating during an MR imaging examination [7]:

  12 W/kg of extremity over 5 minutes
  8 W/kg in any gram of tissue in head or torso
    over 5 minutes

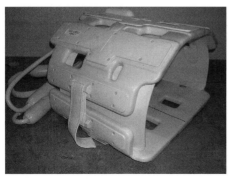

Figure 6 USA Instruments eight-channel torso phased-array receive-only coil used for hip and pelvis imaging.

  4 W/kg of whole body over 15 minutes
  3 W/kg of head over 10 minutes

The SAR that is deposited in tissue is proportional to the duty cycle and radius of tissue, and is exponentially proportional to the magnet field strength and flip angle [8,9]. This is demonstrated in the equation:

$$SAR \propto D\theta^2 (B_0)^2 R$$

where D = duty cycle, θ = flip angle, B_0 = magnetic field, and R = radius of tissue

For a given duty cycle, flip angle, and radius of tissue imaged, the SAR at 3T relative to the SAR at 1.5T is demonstrated in the equation:

$$SAR_{3T} \propto \left(2 \times B_{0(1.5T)}\right)^2 = 4 \times SAR\ 1.5\ T$$

By the first equation, one can see that SAR is worsened with higher duty cycles (shorter TRs and more RF pulses [ie, FSE]). Therefore, SAR effects by sequence type can be summated: FSE > spin echo (SE) > gradient echo (GRE).

Also, larger body parts are subject to more SAR (eg, knee > ankle).

Several techniques can be used to reduce SAR substantially. First and foremost is the use of dedicated transmit-receive surface coils or extremity coils. This markedly reduces the amount of body tissue that is exposed to RF waves, and thereby, reduces SAR. For phased-array receive-only coils, exploiting the reduced duty cycle advantage of parallel imaging achieves a similar effect.

Technical advances have helped to mitigate SAR. Hyperechoes on Siemens systems (Siemens Medical Solutions USA, Malvern, Pennsylvania), described as echoes of echoes, is a novel design of refocusing pulses, which in essence, reduces the effective flip angle and RF deposition [10,11]. Tailored RF, used by GE systems, uses a similar technique. For instance, for an FSE sequence, typically a SAR-intensive scan, lower flip angles are used for refocusing pulses that encode the peripheral lines of k-space. Because SAR depends on the square of the flip angle, any reduction in the flip angle can have powerful ameliorating effects on SAR.

A simple technique for decreasing SAR is to increase the TR value for a given sequence. This decreases the duty cycle of a given sequence by increasing cooling time between repetition pulses. For a given ETL or turbo factor in a fast spin or turbo spin echo technique, doubling the TR effectively decreases the SAR by two. Table 2 shows an example of the effect of TR on a coronal T2-weighted fat-saturated FSE sequence in the knee using an ETL of 10.

Decreasing the ETL (FSE) or turbo factor (TSE) reduces SAR by decreasing the number of 180° RF

Table 2: **Effect of repetition time on specific absorption rate**

TR (ms)	2000	2500	3000	3500	4000
SAR (W/kg)	2.2	1.8	1.5	1.3	1.1

Calculated SAR for different TRs of an FSE sequence in the knee using a fixed ETL of 10.

pulses per repetition. An example of the effect of decreasing ETL on SAR for a coronal T2-weighted FSE sequence of the knee with a TR of 3850 milliseconds is shown in Table 3.

Alternating SAR-intensive sequences with SAR-friendly sequences will help to reduce overall SAR and builds in "cooling time" in an MR imaging examination. For instance, if one had a sequence order as follows:

Sequence 1: FSE
Sequence 2: FSE
Sequence 3: FSE
Sequence 4: SE
Sequence 5: GRE

And knowing that SAR decreases in this order: FSE > SE > GRE [1], the sequence order could be readjusted as follows:

Sequence 1: FSE
Sequence 2: SE
Sequence 3: FSE
Sequence 4: GRE
Sequence 5: FSE

In addition, using parallel imaging techniques can provide another means of reducing SAR effectively. By decreasing the duty cycle in the form of a decreased number of phase-encoding steps, SAR can be decreased. The inherent decrease in SNR can be compensated for by the higher SNR at 3T.

Parallel imaging

Parallel imaging is a technique that uses spatial data that are derived from phased-array coil elements to construct a portion of k-space [12–16]. By using coil elements to supply k-space data, the burden of filling lines of k-space with individually acquired phase gradients is diminished, which decreases the duty cycle of the scan. The end result is a decrease in scan time and—equally important at 3T—a decrease in SAR because of the reduced number of RF pulses that is transmitted to the patient.

Two basic techniques of parallel imaging have been developed; the major manufacturers of MR imaging systems use modified versions of one or both techniques. Simultaneous acquisition of spatial harmonics (SMASH) and sensitivity encoding (SENSE) are two different approaches to parallel imaging [12,14,15]. With SMASH, only a fraction of the lines of k-space is filled with the phase-encoding gradient, whereas the remaining unfilled k-space data are filled by individual coil elements. The final k-space construct is used to create an image. Conversely, with SENSE, each coil element obtains an aliased image (by undersampling k-space or sampling a smaller FOV). These aliased images are combined with an undersampled or decreased FOV k-space acquired with phase-encoding gradients. All of the aliased images are combined mathematically to create an image.

To date, GE's ASSET (array spatial sensitivity encoding technique) and Philips' SENSE use variations of the sensitivity encoding technique of parallel imaging. Siemens' IPAT (Integrated Parallel Acquisition Techniques) combines variations and modifications of SMASH and SENSE.

Parallel imaging can be applied at varying degrees to reduce scan times by factors of two, four, eight, and so forth; this depends on the capabilities of the MR imaging system and the number of coil and receiver channels. The degree of time reduction is referred to as the acceleration factor.

For instance, if a particular coronal sequence of the pelvis is designed for a 512 (phase) × 256 (frequency) matrix, a conventional MR imaging acquisition requires 256 separate phase-encoding steps. By applying parallel imaging with an acceleration factor of two, the number of actual phase-encoding steps is reduced to 128; this reduces the scan time by one half (Fig. 7).

The use of parallel imaging comes at a cost, however. There is a decrease in overall SNR that is proportional to the square root of the acceleration factor ($SNR_{Parallel} \propto 1/\sqrt{\text{acceleration factor}}$). For example, by using an acceleration factor of two, one would expect a decrease in SNR of 40%, whereas by using an acceleration factor of four, one would expect a decrease in SNR of 50%.

Because of the increased signal with 3T scanners, the decrease in SNR that is expected with parallel imaging is compensated. In addition, by decreasing the duty cycle, parallel imaging's SAR-friendliness makes 3T and parallel imaging a perfect marriage [16]. The author's practice uses two parallel-imaging compatible coils for musculoskeletal applications: the MRI Devices eight-channel phased-array

Table 3: **Effect of echo train length on specific absorption rate**

ETL	10	15	20	25
SAR (W/kg)	1.1	1.6	2.0	2.5

Different calculated SAR values for varying ETLs for a coronal FSE sequence in the knee using a fixed TR of 3850.

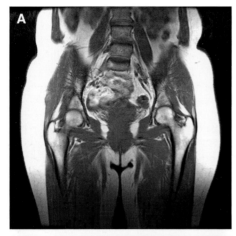

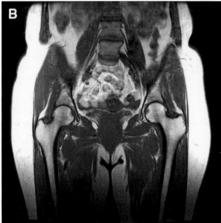

Figure 7 Parallel imaging in the pelvis using the USA Instruments eight-channel phased-array coil. (*A*) Coronal FSE T1-weighted sequence without ASSET with a scan time of 2:56. (*B*) Coronal FSE T1-weighted sequence with ASSET with a scan time of 1:32 and no perceptible loss in SNR.

knee coil (see Fig. 2B) and the USA Instruments eight-channel phased-array torso coil (see Fig. 6). This allows us to achieve an acceleration factor of two with several of our knee, pelvis, and hip sequences. By using an acceleration factor of two in our coronal pelvis sequences, there is no perceptible loss in SNR (see Fig. 7).

In the upcoming months, it is expected that more phased-array coils for other joints will be available and that there will be an increase in the number of channels per coil.

Susceptibility artifact

Metallic hardware in orthopedic imaging notoriously introduces susceptibility artifact; the degree of artifact worsens at higher magnetic field strengths [17]. At 3T, a shortening of T2 and T2* occurs that results in greater signal loss and geometric distortion. In addition, specifically for orthopedic imaging, chemically selective fat-saturation techniques often are markedly inhomogeneous or fail altogether (Fig. 8).

With knee imaging, the most common metallic hardware are anterior cruciate ligament (ACL) graft fixation screws, which often are located far enough from the intra-articular structures so that diagnostic problems rarely arise (see Fig. 8). Most often, the heterogeneous fat saturation limits the assessment of the adjacent bone marrow. In the shoulder, there are occasional diagnostic problems with susceptibility artifact in the rotator cuff tendons after rotator cuff repair. Metallic hardware is encountered less often in the other joints; however, certain techniques can be used to reduce the degree of susceptibility when metal implants are encountered [18–21].

Lengthening ETLs or turbo factors in FSE or TSE sequences decreases susceptibility by the application of additional 180° refocusing pulses [6]; however, increasing ETL comes with a SAR penalty that has to be considered. Increasing bandwidth diminishes susceptibility artifact by decreasing the echo sampling time and minimizing the degree of T2* decay; however, increasing bandwidth decreases SNR as demonstrated by the equation:

$$SNR = K \cdot (VxVyVz) \cdot \sqrt{(NxNyNex/BW)}$$

or

$$SNR \propto \sqrt{1/BW}$$

K = constant, Vx = voxel size in x direction, Vy = voxel size in y direction, Vz = voxel size in z direction, Nx = number of frequency encoding steps, Ny = number of phase encoding steps, Nex = number of excitations, BW = bandwidth

Therefore, by doubling the bandwidth, the SNR is decreased by 40%.

Decreasing the echo time (TE) is another technique to reduce susceptibility. This addresses the T2* and T2 shortening effects at 3T; however, in FSE techniques, the effective TE needs to be adjusted in the context of a long ETL to avoid blurring. In addition, for optimal T2 weighting, decreasing the TE beyond a certain point diminishes contrast-to-noise; therefore, careful consideration for the optimum TE is required.

Decreasing voxel sizes also diminishes susceptibility. By increasing spatial resolution and decreasing slice thickness, a smaller voxel size is achieved. This diminishes the degree of intravoxel dephasing that occurs with metal hardware. The added SNR of 3T compensates for the decrease in SNR from the small voxel size.

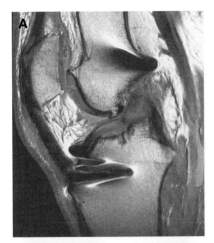

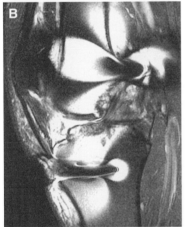

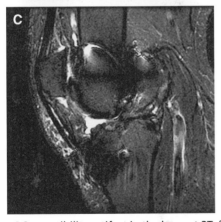

Figure 8 Susceptibility artifact in the knee at 3T. (*A*) A sagittal FSE proton density image of the knee in a patient with ACL graft fixation screws in the distal femur and proximal tibia. This image demonstrates local signal loss and geometric distortion without obscuration of intra-articular structures. (*B*) Sagittal T2-weighted FSE image with chemically selective fat saturation in the same patient demonstrating heterogeneous signal and obscuration of marrow signal. (*C*) Sagittal STIR image in the same patient resulting in more homogenous fat suppression, but with a loss of SNR.

Interesting technical manipulations of the Z-gradient, slice-select RF pulse also have susceptibility reducing capabilities [21,22].

One final option is to use short T1 inversion recovery (STIR) sequences as a substitute for chemically selective fat-saturated T2-weighted images [23]. This improves the homogeneity of fat saturation markedly, but SNR is compromised (see Fig. 8).

Chemical shift artifact

Chemical shift artifact is an issue that must be addressed on musculoskeletal MR images at all field strengths [24]. At 3T, the effects of chemical shift are more pronounced than they are at lower field strengths. An understanding of the factors that determine chemical shift, and techniques to ameliorate these artifacts will dispel any trepidation about imaging at 3T.

The precessional frequency difference between fat protons and water protons is doubled at 3T relative to 1.5T. For instance, at 3T fat precesses 448 Hz faster than water protons; at 1.5T the difference is 224 Hz [25,26]. This results in double the chemical shift artifact at 3T. In the knee, this may become an issue in nonfat-saturated sequences if the artifact becomes superimposed on the menisci or articular cartilage and mimics or obscures pathology.

To counteract the worsened chemical shift, the receiver bandwidth can be increased (Fig. 9). By increasing the bandwidth, the number of frequencies sampled per pixel is increased. Therefore, if there is a shift in frequencies because of chemical shift, fewer pixels are involved and there is a decrease in the perceived size of the chemical shift. For instance, for a 256 frequency matrix and a ± 16-kHz bandwidth, 32,000 Hz are sampled over 256 pixels. This equates to roughly 125 Hz per pixel. Therefore, if there is a chemical shift of 448 Hz, this involves mismapping fat protons by 448 Hz/125 Hz per pixel or 3.58 pixels. For the same matrix, if the bandwidth is doubled to ± 32 kHz, 64,000 Hz would be sampled over 256 pixels, which would result in 64,000/256 or 250 Hz/pixel. A chemical shift of 448 Hz would cause a mismapping of fat protons by 448 Hz/250 Hz per pixel or 1.79 pixels. This is demonstrated in the following:

For a 256 frequency resolution:

±16 kHz bandwidth = 32,000 Hz = 32,000/ 256 or 125 Hz/pixel
Chemical shift = 448/125 or 3.58 pixels
±32 kHz bandwidth = 64,000 Hz = 64,000/ 256 or 250 Hz/pixel
Chemical shift = 448/250 or 1.79 pixels

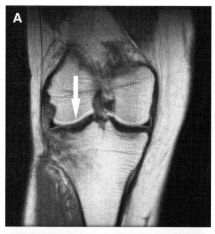

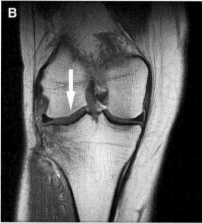

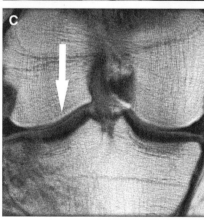

Figure 9 Chemical shift artifact in the knee at 3T demonstrated on coronal FSE T1-weighted images. (*A*) T1-weighted image with a 15-cm FOV and 10-kHz receiver bandwidth demonstrates chemical shift at the lateral femoral condyle (*arrow*). (*B*) T1-weighted image with a 15-cm FOV and 35-kHz receiver bandwidth demonstrates a reduction in the degree of chemical shift (*arrow*). (*C*) T1-weighted image with a 7-cm FOV and 10-kHz receiver bandwidth demonstrates a perceived reduction in the degree of chemical shift that is due to the decrease in pixel size (*arrow*).

When increasing the bandwidth, one should keep in mind the inherent loss of SNR as described in the equation:

$$SNR \propto \sqrt{1/BW}$$

Another technique is to decrease the pixel size and maintain the receiver bandwidth and frequency resolution. To achieve this, a smaller FOV is required (see Fig. 9). This results in a perceived smaller distance of chemical shift. For instance, at ± 16 kHz bandwidth, a 256 matrix with a 16-cm FOV results in a 3.58 pixel chemical shift. Each pixel measures 160 mm/256 pixels or 0.625 mm. The total chemical shift distance would be 0.625 mm/pixel × 3.58 pixels or 2.24 mm. If the FOV were decreased to 8 cm, each pixel would measure 80 mm/256 pixels or 0.31 mm; the total chemical shift distance would be 0.31 mm/pixel × 3.58 pixels or 1.12 mm. This technique is not of practical usefulness because of the introduction of aliasing or wrap-around artifact.

Chemical shift artifact usually does not cause a diagnostic dilemma in the shoulder, elbow, wrist, and hip. Most assessments of the rotator cuff and glenoid labrum involve T2-weighted fat-saturated sequences, which eliminates the issue of chemical shift. Furthermore, T1-weighted sequences usually provide information about marrow lesions (contusions, cysts, fractures), soft tissue masses, hematomas or hemorrhage, loose bodies, and muscle atrophy. Chemical shift rarely factors into these assessments.

In the ankle, potential chemical shift–related diagnostic problems may arise at the talar dome cartilage; however, fat-saturated sequences generally are used for cartilage assessment, which eliminates any chemical shift artifact. In addition, T1 sequences usually provide information about marrow lesions (contusions, osteochondral lesions, fractures), and the use of a routine receiver bandwidth of 41 kHz almost completely eliminates any perceptible chemical shift while maintaining adequate SNR (Fig. 10).

Pulsation artifact

Pulsation or flow artifact worsens at higher field strengths [27,28]. In the knee, the popliteal vessels may result in artifact that obscures the posterior horns of the menisci, especially on sagittal sequences (Fig. 11). Several techniques may be used to diminish pulsation artifact (see Fig. 11). Application of saturation bands superiorly, inferiorly, or in both locations may help to decrease pulsation; however, this may result in prolonged scan times and increased SAR.

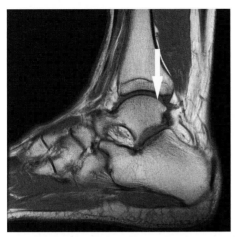

Figure 10 Sagittal T1-weighted image of the ankle with a receiver bandwidth of 41 kHz demonstrates little appreciable chemical shift artifact at the talar dome (*arrow*).

In addition, choosing the correct phase-encoding direction is beneficial in directing the pulsation artifacts over noncrucial structures. For instance, on a sagittal knee sequence, choosing a superior-to-inferior phase direction ensures that pulsation artifacts are propagated along the posterior soft tissues, whereas, choosing an anterior-to-posterior phase direction places the artifacts over the internal structures of the knee.

Using the flow compensation feature to achieve gradient moment nulling of the first order may alleviate pulsation artifacts [29]; however, this usually results in prolongation of the minimum TE, which may become an issue for T1- or proton density–weighted images.

Truncation artifact

Truncation artifact is a well-known artifact that occurs commonly at the interface between low- and high-signal structures [30], such as the vertebral bodies and cerebrospinal fluid (CSF) on a sagittal T2-weighted sequence. At 3T, because of the higher SNR of all tissues, this phenomenon also becomes apparent in extremity imaging. In the knee, truncation may occur at the interface of bone and joint fluid. To correct truncation, an increase in phase resolution is required.

Dielectric resonance (field focusing)

At 3T, the Larmor frequency is approximately 128 MHz. As a result, the wavelengths of RF pulses are decreased proportionately compared with 1.5T scanners. In addition, the dielectric constant of tissues increases at higher field strengths. A higher dielectric constant effectively results in slower

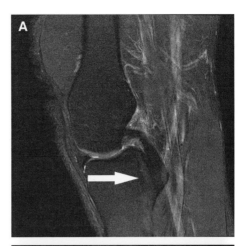

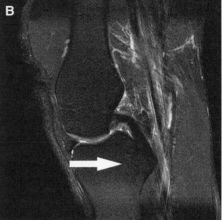

Figure 11 Sagittal T2-weighted FSE images with fat saturation of the knee. (*A*) Pulsation artifact is seen over the posterior aspect of the medial tibial plateau (*arrow*) in this image without saturation bands or flow compensation. (*B*) The degree of pulsation artifact is diminished (*arrow*) in the same patient when superior and inferior saturation bands within the edges of the field of view are applied, and flow compensation is applied in the frequency direction.

electromagnetic waves with shorter wavelengths. As a result of the shorter wavelengths of the RF pulses and higher dielectric constant of tissue, there is an increased incidence of standing waves. The effect is interference with the B_1 field [31,32]. The end result is an inhomogeneous image or an image with a bright center and hypointense periphery. Dielectric pads are available and can be placed next to the patient to correct this artifact; dielectric effect rarely is a problem in extremity imaging.

T1 relaxation times

The effect of higher field strength on T1 relaxation times is a component of 3T imaging that requires

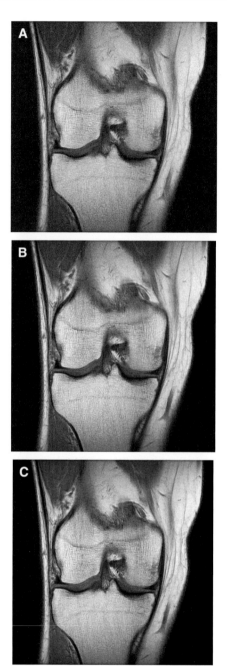

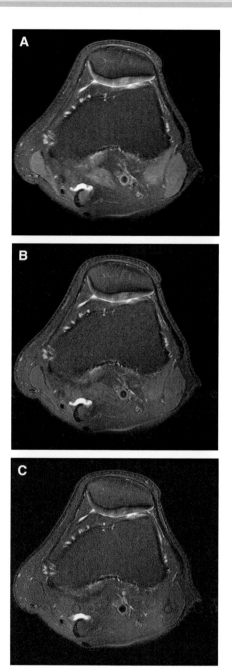

Figure 12 Coronal FSE T1-weighted images of the knee at 3T with an ETL of 3 using various TR values. (*A*) A TR of 250 milliseconds and a TE of 9 milliseconds demonstrate overall slightly diminished SNR and decreased muscle signal, but adequate contrast between various tissues. (*B*) A TR of 500 milliseconds and a TE of 9 milliseconds demonstrate excellent contrast between various tissues and an improvement in overall SNR. (*C*) A TR of 1000 milliseconds and a TE of 9 milliseconds show only minimal changes in signal contrast of various tissues compared with smaller TR values.

Figure 13 Axial FSE T2-weighted images of the knee using an ETL of 12 and various TE values. (*A*) Image obtained with a TR of 4150 milliseconds and a TE of 35 milliseconds shows good cartilage–fluid contrast and high cartilage signal. (*B*) Image obtained with a TR of 4150 milliseconds and a TE of 55 milliseconds demonstrates good cartilage–fluid contrast and slightly lower overall cartilage signal. (*C*) Image obtained with a TR of 4150 milliseconds and a TE of 75 milliseconds demonstrates good cartilage–fluid contrast and slightly lower overall tissue signal.

consideration. It is well documented that the T1 relaxation time for most tissues increases with increasing field strength [33–36]. As a result, the TR for T1-weighted sequences needs to be prolonged to optimize T1 differences between tissues. In addition, for proton density and T2-weighted images, TRs also need to be prolonged to eliminate T1 weighting.

A recent study demonstrated the T1 times of tissues of the knee at 3T compared with at 1.5T [36]. Of note are the T1 times for subcutaneous fat and marrow fat; at 3T these are increased by 22% and 21%, respectively. The T1 time for synovial fluid also is increased by 21%. This has implications for T2-weighted or proton density–weighted images, which require an increase in TR to eliminate any residual T1 weighting.

The increase in TR results in longer scan times, but has the advantages of decreasing SAR and allowing more slices per scan. The optimal TR value for T1-weighted images is not a complicated issue in the extremities, because the prolongation of T1 values seems to be similar for all tissue types, unlike for the brain. Therefore, extending TR values by at least 20% over 1.5T parameters should account for the 20% average prolongation in T1 times. In reality, however, a wide range of TRs can accomplish T1-weighting of diagnostic value as demonstrated in Fig. 12, which shows excellent tissue contrast at varying TR values.

T2 decay times

Although not as dramatic as the effect on T1 relaxation, higher field strengths shorten the T2 decay times of various tissues [33–36]. As a result, TE times need to be shortened on T1-, T2-, and proton density–weighted images to compensate for the decrease in T2 and T2*. In addition, a theoretic increase in image blurring may occur with FSE sequences, because the lower-signal, longer TE echoes fill the peripheral lines of k-space. Susceptibility artifacts also may worsen as a result of the shortening of T2*.

Gold and colleagues [36] demonstrated T2 times for various tissues around the knee at 3T and 1.5T. In that study, however, there was an improvement in the tissue contrast between joint fluid and articular cartilage for various TR values compared with at 1.5T. Although there was a greater effect on T2 shortening for synovial fluid (36.6%) than there was for cartilage (12.3%), the actual T2 value for synovial fluid remained high (767 milliseconds) relative to the TE values that were used in T2-weighted images. This results in a maintenance of high signal for fluid at 3T and a relative decrease in signal in articular cartilage, which maximizes the contrast between the two tissues. Theoretically, this improves the visibility of cartilage surface lesions. TE times should be adjusted, however, to accommodate for the relative loss in cartilage signal at 3T. Despite this theoretic concern, a range of TE times may be used on T2-weighted images to achieve high diagnostic value (Fig. 13).

Summary

As 3T MR imaging systems become more widespread in the clinical realm, a full understanding of the opportunities for image improvement and the limitations in the applications of the signal gain is needed. It is clear that even with current coil technology, much of the gain in signal can be harnessed effectively; however, continued coil development is necessary to realize the full potential of 3T, especially with the wonderful synergy that can be achieved with the use of parallel imaging and multiple-channel phased-array extremity coils.

Furthermore, despite the theoretic imaging challenges at higher field strengths (eg, susceptibility, chemical shift, SAR, pulsation, T1 time prolongation, and T2 time shortening), the techniques and methods that were discussed above can eliminate any obstacles to clinical imaging. This creates excellent opportunities to improve image quality, spatial resolution, and diagnostic accuracy in the musculoskeletal system. From the author's experience, the superb image quality has impressed referring orthopedic surgeons, and the reduction in scan time has resulted in greater patient satisfaction and reduced anxiety.

References

[1] Parker DL, Gullberg GT. Signal-to-noise efficiency in magnetic resonance imaging. Med Phys 1990;17:250–7.

[2] Edelman RE, Hesselink JR, Zlatkin MB. Clinical magnetic resonance imaging. 2nd edition. Philadelphia: WB Saunders; 1996.

[3] Ciobanu L, Webb AG, Pennington CH. Magnetic resonance imaging of biological cells. Prog Nuc Magn Reson Spect 2003;42:69–93.

[4] Sotgiu A, Hyde JS. High-order coils as transmitters for NMR imaging. Magn Reson Med 1986; 3:55–62.

[5] Hoult DI, Chen CN, Sank VJ. Quadrature detection in the laboratory frame. Magn Reson Med 1984;1:339–53.

[6] Roemer PB, Edelstein WA, Hayes CE, et al. The NMR phased array. Magn Reson Med 1990; 16:192–225.

[7] US Food and Drug Administration. Center for Devices and Radiological Health. Guidance for

Industry and FDA Staff. Criteria for significant risk investigations of magnetic resonance diagnostic devices. Rockville (MD): US Food and Drug Administration; 2003.

[8] Bottomley PA, Redington RW, Edelstein WA, et al. Estimating radiofrequency power deposition in body NMR imaging. Magn Reson Med 1985;2:336–49.

[9] Price RR. The AAPM/RSNA physics tutorial for residents. MR imaging safety considerations. Radiological Society of North America. Radiographics 1999;19:1641–51.

[10] Hennig J, Scheffler K. Hyperechoes. Magn Reson Med 2001;46:6–12.

[11] Prost JE, Wehrli FW, Drayer B, et al. SAR reduced pulse sequences. Magn Reson Imaging 1988;6:125–30.

[12] Sodickson DK, Manning WJ. Simultaneous acquisition of spatial harmonics (SMASH): fast imaging with radiofrequency coil arrays. Magn Reson Med 1997;38:591–603.

[13] Sodickson DK, McKenzie CA. A generalized approach to parallel magnetic resonance imaging. Med Phys 2001;28:1629–43.

[14] Sodickson DK, Griswold MA, Jakob PM. SMASH imaging. Magn Reson Imaging Clin N Am 1999;7:237–54.

[15] Pruessman KP, Weiger M, Scheidegger MB, et al. SENSE: sensitivity encoding for fast MRI. Magn Reson Med 1999;42:952–62.

[16] Pruessmann KP. Parallel imaging at high field strength: synergies and joint potential. Top Magn Reson Imaging 2004;15:237–44.

[17] Abduljalil AM, Robitaille PM. Macroscopic susceptibility in ultra high field MRI. J Comput Assist Tomogr 1999;23:832–41.

[18] Herold T, Caro WC, Heers G, et al. Influence of sequence type on the extent of the susceptibility artifact in MRI–a shoulder specimen study after suture anchor repair. Rofo 2005;176:1296–301.

[19] Petersilge CA. Evaluation of the postoperative spine: reducing hardware artifacts during magnetic resonance imaging. Semin Musculoskelet Radiol 2000;4:293–7.

[20] Port JD, Pomper MG. Quantification and minimization of magnetic susceptibility artifacts on GRE images. J Comput Assist Tomogr 2000;24:958–64.

[21] Cho ZH, Ro YM. Reduction of susceptibility artifact in gradient-echo imaging. Magn Reson Med 1992;23:193–200.

[22] Stenger VA, Boada FE, Noll DC. Three-dimensional tailored RF pulses for the reduction of susceptibility artifacts in $T(*)(2)$-weighted functional MRI. Magn Reson Med 2000;44:525–31.

[23] Viano AM, Gronemeyer SA, Haliloglu M, et al. Improved MR imaging for patients with metallic implants. Magn Reson Imaging 2000;18:287–95.

[24] Peh WC, Chan JH. Artifacts in musculoskeletal magnetic resonance imaging: identification and correction. Skeletal Radiol 2001;30:179–91.

[25] Sakurai K, Fujita N, Murakami T, et al. Effects of sampling bandwidth in MR imaging. Nippon Igaku Hoshasen Gakkai Zasshi 1990;50:910–7.

[26] Hood MN, Ho VB, Smirniotopoulos JG, et al. Chemical shift: the artifact and clinical tool revisited. Radiographics 1999;19:357–71.

[27] Lenk S, Ludescher B, Martirosan P, et al. 3T high-resolution MR imaging of carpal ligaments and TFCC. Rofo 2004;176:664–7.

[28] Naganawa S, Koshikawa T, Nakamura T, et al. Comparison of flow artifacts between 2D-FLAIR and 3D-FLAIR sequences at 3T. Eur Radiol 2004;14:1901–8.

[29] Hinks RS, Constable RT. Gradient moment nulling in fast spin echo. Magn Reson Med 1994;32:698–706.

[30] Lufkin RB, Pusey E, Stark DD, et al. Boundary artifact due to truncation errors in MR imaging. AJR Am J Roentgenol 1986;147:1283–7.

[31] Crozier S, Brereton IM, Zelaya FO, et al. Sample-induced RF perturbations in high-field, high-resolution NMR spectroscopy. J Magn Reson 1997;126:39–47.

[32] Alsop DC, Connick TJ, Mizsei G. A spiral volume coil for improved RF field homogeneity at high static magnetic field strength. Magn Reson Med 1998;40:49–54.

[33] Jezzard P, Duewell S, Balaban RS. MR relaxation times in human brain: measurement at 4 T. Radiology 1996;199:773–9.

[34] Gomori JM, Grossman RI, Yu-Ip C, et al. NMR relaxation times of blood: dependence on field strength, oxidation state, and cell integrity. J Comput Assist Tomogr 1987;11:684–90.

[35] Cremillieux Y, Ding S, Dunn JF. High-resolution in vivo measurements of transverse relaxation times in rats at 7 Tesla. Magn Reson Med 1998;39:285–90.

[36] Gold GE, Han E, Stainsby J, et al. Musculoskeletal MRI at 3.0T: relaxation times and image contrast. AJR Am J Roentgenol 2004;183:343–51.

MAGNETIC
RESONANCE
IMAGING CLINICS

Magn Reson Imaging Clin N Am (2006) 41–62

3T MR Imaging of the Musculoskeletal System (Part II): Clinical Applications

R. Richard Ramnath MD

With the rapid development of 3T MR imaging systems, the theoretic applications in the musculoskeletal system are now a reality. The gain in the signal-to-noise ratio (SNR) can be applied in multiple fashions to improve image quality or to improve scan time. By choosing to improve image quality by increasing in-plane resolution or decreasing slice thickness, the potential for demonstrating the intrinsic structures of joints in greater detail is a tantalizing option. With increased signal and higher spatial resolutions, the potential for improved diagnostic accuracy is obvious.

If MR imaging on current conventional field strengths delivers satisfactory diagnostic accuracies, then the role for higher field strengths in the diagnosis of joint disease should be scrutinized to justify the cost of investing in 3T systems. The evaluation of intra-articular pathology, such as meniscal pathology in the knee or rotator cuff tears in the shoulder, has been successful with routine MR imaging. In each of the six major joints, many of the smaller ligamentous and cartilaginous structures evade adequate evaluation on 1.5T systems using routine nonarthrographic images. With the use of 3T systems, one can enhance the SNR, spatial resolution, and contrast-to-noise ratio (CNR) of these structures, which makes them more discernible and amenable to proper radiologic assessment. In turn, an improvement in the diagnosis of pathologic conditions will be augmented.

Over the past 2 years, the author's practice has achieved great success in applying 3T systems to

Neuroskeletal Imaging, 1344 South Apollo Boulevard, Suite 406, Melbourne, FL 32901, USA
E-mail address: rramnath@neuroskeletal.com

1064-9689/06/$ – see front matter © 2006 Elsevier Inc. All rights reserved.
mri.theclinics.com
doi:10.1016/j.mric.2006.01.003

musculoskeletal imaging. The ligamentous and cartilaginous structures have been elucidated in better detail, and diagnoses that would have been ambiguous in years past have been made more confidently. Many of the author's referring orthopedic surgeons have appreciated the improvement in image quality and diagnostic assessment, and several request only 3T MR images for their patients. With a little diligence and minor adjustments to protocol parameters, impressive high-resolution 3T images can be produced easily.

Knee

With certain structures of the knee, the ability to evaluate pathology is excellent with conventional MR field strengths. With other areas of the knee, improvements in diagnostic abilities are needed, which opens the door for the high-resolution, high-signal capabilities of 3T systems.

Menisci

The ability to detect meniscal tears has a broad range of accuracies in the literature; however, more recent studies showed superb results. The evaluation of menisci with MR imaging has long been shown to be a highly accurate endeavor with sensitivities ranging from 40% to 100% [1–8], specificities ranging from 72% to 100% [1–6], and accuracies ranging from 75% to 96% [1,5,9–11].

Several articles in the orthopedic literature suggested equal or better diagnostic accuracy with the use of a proper physical examination [5,10,12,13]. Kocabey and colleagues [12] recently reported equivalent diagnostic accuracies of a physical examination by a skilled orthopedic surgeon in the detection of medial and lateral meniscal tears. The article further advocated only obtaining an MR image in "more complicated and confusing" cases. Muellner and colleagues [5] demonstrated a 95% accuracy, 97% sensitivity, and 87% specificity for the detection of meniscal tears with clinical examination alone. Stanitski [13] found a highly negative correlation between arthroscopic and MR imaging findings and stated that "magnetic resonance imaging diagnoses added little guidance to patient management and at times provided spurious information".

With the advent of 3T MR imaging, the potential for greater spatial resolution and higher SNR could be used effectively to improve upon the accuracy of 1.5T systems or at least improve diagnostic confidence, and further illustrate to orthopedic surgeons the value of MR imaging in the routine assessment of meniscal pathology. In the author's practice, meniscal tears of all types are demonstrated beautifully. Fig. 1 illustrates various meniscal tear types,

including a horizontal tear with a corresponding arthroscopic image, a radial tear, a peripheral vertical tear, and a case of simultaneous bicompartmental bucket-handle tears [14].

Cruciate ligaments

The cruciate ligaments, and more specifically the anterior cruciate ligament (ACL), have been studied extensively with MR imaging. Many investigators demonstrated terrific success in the diagnosis of acute and subacute ACL tears [15–21]. These studies showed sensitivities of 92% to 100%, specificities of 85% to 100%, and accuracies of 89% to 100%. Fig. 2 demonstrates a full-thickness tear of the ACL at 3T with arthroscopic correlation. The assessment of partial and chronic tears of the posterior cruciate ligament (PCL) and the ACL has been disappointing, however [22–26]. For partial ACL tears, a sensitivity range of 40% to 75% and specificity range of 62% to 89% have been published. It is questionable whether higher field-strength systems will improve on current diagnostic accuracies in assessing partial tears. There is a role for higher field strengths in the evaluation of partial tears given the low accuracy at 1.5T.

Although an uncommon injury, tears of the posterior cruciate ligament are evaluated well on current magnet strengths [27,28], and any added improvement with higher field strength systems is unlikely.

Articular cartilage

The assessment of the articular cartilage of the knee has had varied success with MR imaging, depending on the sequences that were used. For all cartilage defect grades, sensitivities range from 33% to 94% [29–38], specificities rage from 89% to 99% [29–38], and accuracies range from 73% to 98% [29,31–38]. The diagnostic accuracy for high-grade lesions is greater than for low-grade lesions [31]. In one study, the detection of grade 1 lesions resulted in sensitivities of 53% to 73%, specificities of 65% to 75%, and accuracies of 62% to 70%, depending on whether gradient echo or fast spin echo (FSE) techniques were used [39]. For grade 2 lesions, sensitivities were 43% to 60%, specificities were 92%, and accuracies were 83% to 86% [39]. In another study, the sensitivity and specificity for grades 1 and 2 lesions were 75% and 94%, respectively, and were 80% and 99%, respectively, for grades 3 and 4 lesions [40]. Another study that evaluated only grades 3 and 4 lesions showed a sensitivity of 83%, a specificity of 97%, and an accuracy of 93% [41]. Similar differences in accuracy for low- and high-grade lesions were found in the study by Macarini and colleagues [42].

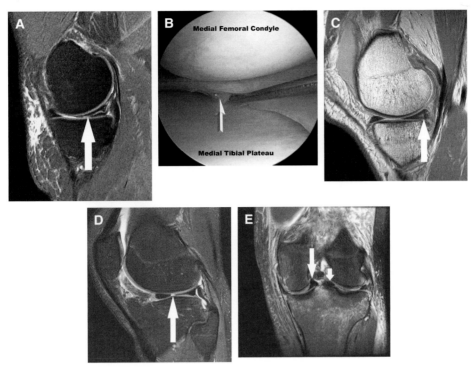

Figure 1 Various meniscal tears demonstrated on images from a 3T MR imaging system. (*A*) Horizontal cleavage tear of the body and posterior horn of the medial meniscus extending to the free edge (*arrow*) seen on a sagittal fast spin echo (FSE) T2-weighted fat saturated image. (*B*) Arthroscopic image of the same patient shows the surgical probe within the tear at the free margin of the medial meniscus (*arrow*). (Courtesy of LeRoy Gurganious, MD, Melbourne, FL.) (*C*) A peripheral vertical tear of the posterior horn of the medial meniscus that extends to the inferior articular surface (*arrow*) is demonstrated on a sagittal FSE PD image. The diagnosis was confirmed at arthroscopy. (*D*) A radial tear of the body of the lateral meniscus (*arrow*) is seen on a sagittal FSE T2-weighted fat-saturated image. (*E*) Bicompartmental bucket-handle tears of the medial (*long arrow*) and lateral (*short arrow*) menisci as seen on a coronal FSE T2-weighted image.

The improved signal, CNR, and spatial resolution advantages of 3T may improve these deficiencies. One study showed that with improved spatial resolution, the assessment of articular cartilage is improved [43]. In this report, in-plane resolution is optimal at 39 μm, which for a 15-cm field of view (FOV) study equals a 3846 × 3846 matrix [43]. Suboptimal in-plane resolution was demonstrated with 600-μm voxel sizes or a 250 × 250 matrix at 15-cm FOV [43]. The in-plane resolution of 39 μm was obtained in cadaveric specimens at 7.1T. This might not be achievable for practical clinical use, but any improvement in resolution that could be afforded by a higher field strength system would be advantageous.

In addition to the advantage of improved spatial resolution at 3T, a recent study demonstrated a greater CNR between articular cartilage and joint fluid at 3T, which would assist further in cartilage assessment [44]. The improved contrast-to-noise ratio was seen at a wide range of repetition times (TRs) [44].

Initial studies attempted to compare the efficacy of 3T MR imaging with 1.5T MR imaging in the evaluation of articular cartilage. In 2004, Schroder and colleagues [45] demonstrated an improved efficacy at 3T only for fat-saturated two- and three-dimensional (3D) gradient echo sequences and only in lesion detection, not in lesion size. No improvement was seen at 3T using fat-saturated FSE proton-density (PD) sequences for lesion detection. Surprisingly, for assessing the length and depth of lesions, there was no advantage to any sequence at 3T. One should keep in mind that this study was performed on sheep cadavers.

The same group published data that compared 3T MR imaging with 1.5T MR imaging for cartilage lesion detection, SNR, and CNR using three different sequences. This study demonstrated further the improvement in lesion detection, SNR, and CNR for all sequences on 3T MR imaging [46]. **Fig. 3** illustrates partial- and full-thickness cartilage lesions, including a delamination injury [47].

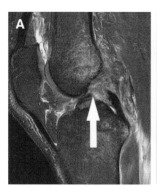 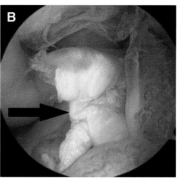

Figure 2 Full-thickness midsubstance ACL rupture. (*A*) Full-thickness ACL tear with a residual distal stump (*arrow*). (*B*) Arthroscopic photograph of the distal ACL stump (*arrow*). (Courtesy of LeRoy Gurganious, MD, Melbourne, FL.)

In recent years, many researchers have focused on the alteration in T2 decay times of articular cartilage as an early indicator of osteoarthritis. T2 time alterations are caused by a combination of proteoglycan content depletion, changes in water content, and increase in collagen content, as well as variations in matrix components in different cartilage layers [48–56]. Although several studies demonstrated successful T2 mapping of articular cartilage using 1.5T systems [54,55], the potential advantage of higher field strengths is undeniable in the ability to increase the signal that is obtained from articular cartilage. The slight decrease in T2 decay times at higher field strengths—estimated at approximately 12% at 3T compared with 1.5T [44]—is unlikely to detract significantly from the accuracy of T2 mapping.

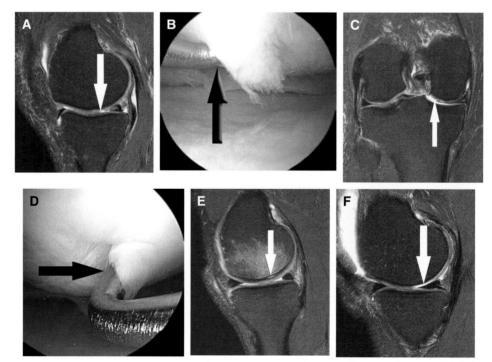

Figure 3 Cartilage lesions demonstrated on 3T MR images. (*A*) Partial-thickness cartilage flap seen at the medial femoral condyle (*arrow*) on a sagittal FSE T2-weighted fat-saturated image. (*B*) Arthroscopic photograph of the same cartilage flap. The arrow points to the surgical probe lifting the flap for better visibility. (*C*) Partial-thickness cartilage defect involving the medial femoral condyle (*arrow*) as demonstrated on a coronal FSE T2-weighted fat-saturated image. (*D*) Arthroscopic photograph of the same cartilage defect showing the surgical probe exploring the lesion (*arrow*). (*E*) Delamination injury at the cartilage–bone interface (*arrow*) on a sagittal FSE T2-weighted fat-saturated image. (*F*) Full-thickness cartilage defect overlying the medial femoral condyle (*arrow*) as seen on a sagittal FSE T2-weighted fat-saturated image. (Arthroscopic photographs are courtesy of LeRoy Gurganious, MD, Melbourne, FL).

The posterolateral corner

The potential improvement in spatial resolution at 3T affords the opportunity to evaluate better the smaller structures of the knee, such as the posterolateral corner. This important anatomic complex prevents varus knee stress and external rotation, and is an important anterior and posterior stabilizer. Posterolateral corner instability contributes to ACL graft reconstruction failure [57]. Therefore, it is important to identify these injuries before surgery.

Several surgical techniques may be used, including primary repair in acute injuries and allograft reconstruction techniques that use anterior tibialis, posterior tibialis, or hamstring tendons for chronic tears or acute tears with insufficient reparable tissue [58–60]. The structures of the posterolateral corner may be amenable to better identification and delineation with higher field strength systems. These structures include the biceps femoris, popliteus tendon, popliteomeniscal fascicles, popliteofibular ligament, fibular collateral ligament, fabellofibular ligament, arcuate ligament, coronary ligament, and lateral third midcapsular ligament. Fig. 4 illustrates a normal popliteofibular ligament.

The posteromedial corner

Recent attention in the orthopedic literature has focused on the structures of the posteromedial corner in terms of contribution to the anatomy and function of the normal knee, and instability patterns as they relate to ACL ruptures and ACL repair [61–63]. These important structures stabilize against anterior and medial subluxation of the tibia and

prevent valgus stress. Injury to the posteromedial corner may occur in the setting of ACL injury [61]. The structures of the posteromedial corner include the posterior horn of the medial meniscus, semimembranosus tendon, posterior oblique ligament, and oblique popliteal ligament. 3T MR imaging has the potential to improve the anatomic delineation of these structures. The exact surgical management for posteromedial corner injury has not been determined.

How it is done

Currently, the author uses the Medical Advances quadrature transmit-receive knee coil with chimney component or the MRI Devices eight-channel receive-only phased-array coil on the GE (General Electric, Milwaukee, Wisconsin) 3T MR imaging system with the high definition (HD) Excite platform. Five sequences are acquired for a total scan time of 15 minutes and 50 seconds in a 30-minute time slot. The following sequences are used: coronal FSE T2 with fat saturation, coronal FSE T1, sagittal FSE PD, sagittal FSE T2 with fat saturation, and axial FSE T2 with fat saturation (Table 1).

The author's main meniscal workhorse sequence is the sagittal FSE PD-weighted sequence. The T2-weighed sequences in all three planes are used to assess articular cartilage, collateral ligaments, cruciate ligaments, and marrow lesions (fractures, contusions, tumors). The coronal T1-weighted sequence is used to evaluate marrow abnormalities (fractures, osteochondral lesions, contusions, tumors) and to provide additional assessment of menisci.

Shoulder

MR imaging has long been used to evaluate pathologic conditions of the shoulder with great success; however, certain anatomic structures have not been served well with conventional MR imaging field strengths.

Rotator cuff

The rotator cuff can be evaluated well on 1.5T systems. Although a wide range of results has been published, more recent reports show excellent detection of full-thickness rotator cuff tears by MR imaging. For full-thickness rotator cuff tears, sensitivities of 56% to 100%, specificities of 69% to 100%, and accuracies of 69% to 97% have been shown [64–81]. Any potential improvement in accuracy on 3T is likely to be slight given the already high degree of sensitivity and specificity. In general, full-thickness rotator cuff tears are elucidated well on 3T MR imaging examinations with excellent anatomic resolution and signal contrast between the fluid within a tear and the involved tendon (Fig. 5).

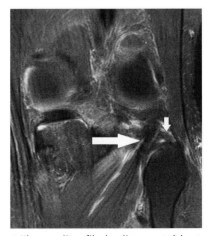

Figure 4 The popliteofibular ligament (*short arrow*) demonstrated on a coronal FSE T2-weighted fat-saturated image that was obtained on a 3T MR imaging system. The popliteus tendon is well demonstrated (*long arrow*).

Table 1:   **3T MR imaging knee protocol**

Parameters	Coronal fat-saturated FSE T2	Coronal FSE T1	Sagittal FSE PD	Sagittal fat-saturated FSE T2	Axial fat-saturated FSE T2
TR (ms)	3925	625	3950	4050	3950
TE (ms)	55	9	10	55	55
ETL	12	3	6	12	12
NEX	2	1	1	2	2
Phase direction	R to L	R to L	S to I	S to I	R to L
FOV (cm)	15	15	16	15	15
Frequency	384	512	512	384	384
Phase	320	384	320	320	320
BW (kHz)	31	41	50	25	31
Slice (mm)	4	4	2	3	4
Gap (mm)	1	1	0.2	1	1
Scan time	3:05	2:17	3:29	3:54	3:05

The protocol is optimized for the MRI Devices knee coil on the GE 3T MR imaging system with the HD Excite platform. *Abbreviations:* BW, bandwidth; ETL, echo train length; FOV, field-of-view; I, inferior; L, left; NEX, number of excitations; R, right; S, superior; TE, echo time; TR, repetition time.

Improved diagnostic confidence with questionable findings and partial tears is highly possible. The ability to detect partial rotator cuff tears is suboptimal with sensitivities of 0% to 83%, specificities of 68% to 97%, and accuracies of 59% to 87% [67,69,73,74,76,79]. Although the diagnosis of partial rotator cuff tears on 3T is straightforward in most cases (Fig. 6), there is an important diagnostic role for MR arthrography, despite the improved SNR of 3T on nonarthrographic images. The author's practice has several cases of full-thickness and partial-thickness tears that would have been missed without MR arthrography (Fig. 7). As was shown previously [79–84] at 1.5T, direct MR arthrography can achieve 100% sensitivity and specificity in the detection of undersurface partial- and full-thickness rotator cuff tears. This suggests that

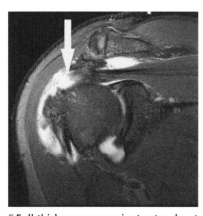

Figure 5 Full-thickness supraspinatus tendon tear (*arrow*) near the attachment to the greater tuberosity is seen on a 3T coronal oblique FSE T2-weighted fat-saturated image. Excellent fluid–tendon contrast is demonstrated.

higher field strength systems may not replace the need for MR arthrography completely, but may decrease the number of ambiguous cases that requires additional arthrographic assessment. Furthermore, the enhanced spatial resolution and signal at 3T can bolster the MR arthrographic images and improve the visibility of tears.

Glenoid labrum and instability

Radiologists' ability to assess the glenoid labrum has been varied at 1.5T, with generally low sensitivities and slightly higher specificities. For all labral pathology, published data include sensitivities of 36% to 78%, specificities of 54% to 100%, and accuracies of 55% to 80% [85–92]. One study showed excellent results with a sensitivity of 98%, a specificity of 89.5%, and an accuracy of 95.7% for detecting tears of the superior labrum [93]. The author's anecdotal experience is that tears and the pathologic signal of the glenoid labrum are seen more easily with 3T systems than with 1.5T systems (Fig. 8).

To improve on the diagnostic ability of 1.5T systems, direct MR arthrography may be used to detect labral pathology, as shown in several reports [83,94–100]. These studies revealed sensitivities of 48% to 100%, specificities of 69% to 100%, and accuracies of 74% to 92%. The use of indirect arthrography also improved the detection of labral pathology with sensitivities of 71% to 91%, specificities of 80% to 85%, and accuracies of 89% to 100% [101,102].

The improved signal, CNR, and spatial resolution advantages of 3T may improve the deficiencies of nonarthrographic MR imaging. One study compared the ability to detect SLAP (superior labrum

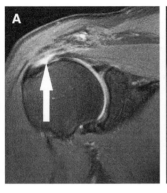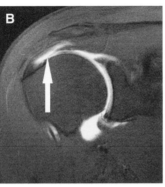

Figure 6 Articular surface partial tear of the supraspinatus tendon is seen well on 3T MR imaging. (*A*) A fluid-filled defect is seen at the articular surface and intrasubstance fibers of the supraspinatus tendon (*arrow*) on a coronal oblique FSE T2-weighted fat-saturated sequence. (*B*) MR arthrographic image confirms the presence of an articular surface partial tear by the extension of contrast into the supraspinatus tendon (*arrow*) as seen on a coronal oblique FSE T1 fat-saturated image.

anterior to posterior) tears using high-field (1.5T) and low-field (0.2 T) systems; sensitivities of 90% and 64% were found with the 1.5T system and the low-field system, respectively [103]. Magee and colleagues [104] also compared patients who were scanned on high-field (1.5T) and low-field (0.2 T) systems; the low-field system failed to demonstrate five labral tears that were shown on the higher field strength. One can conclude that with the gain in SNR on the higher field strength system, diagnostic accuracy is improved. Whether 3T systems will replace the need for direct or indirect arthrography is unclear and is unlikely, because of the advantages of intra-articular distention with MR arthrography. MR arthrography continues to play an important role in the assessment of the glenoid labrum in the author's practice. Several normal or near-normal appearing labra on routine images were diagnosed as being torn with MR arthrography (Fig. 9).

How it is done

The author uses the USA Instruments (Aurora, Ohio) three-channel phased-array receive-only shoulder coil or the MRI Devices eight-channel, phased-array receive-only shoulder coil on the GE 3T MR imaging system with the HD Excite platform. Five sequences are acquired for a total scan time of 14 minutes and 20 seconds in a 30-minute time slot. The following five sequences are used: coronal oblique FSE T2 with fat saturation, coronal oblique FSE T1, sagittal oblique FSE T2 with fat saturation, sagittal oblique FSE T1, and axial FSE T2 with fat saturation (Table 2).

The T2-weighed sequences in the coronal and sagittal planes are used to assess the rotator cuff.

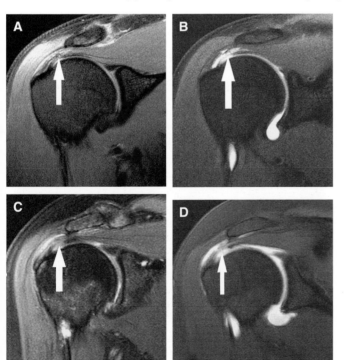

Figure 7 Partial- and full-thickness rotator cuff tears can be found on MR arthrography, but not on routine 3T images. (*A*) Mildly increased signal within the supraspinatus tendon (*arrow*) was interpreted prospectively as tendinopathy on a coronal oblique FSE T2-weighted fat-saturated sequence. (*B*) MR arthrographic image demonstrates an articular surface partial tear by extension of contrast into the supraspinatus tendon (*arrow*) on a coronal oblique FSE T1-weighted fat-saturated sequence. (*C*) Mildly increased signal and contour irregularity was interpreted prospectively as tendinopathy with possible inferior surface fraying (*arrow*) on a coronal oblique FSE T2-weighted fat-saturated sequence. (*D*) MR arthrographic image demonstrates contrast pooling in the subacromial space and confirms a full-thickness tear, likely a microperforation because of the lack of a significant contrast-filled defect (*arrow*) in the supraspinatus tendon.

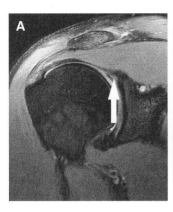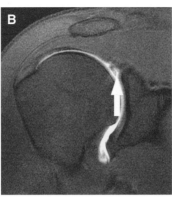

Figure 8 SLAP tears demonstrated at 3T. (*A*) Abnormal signal in the superior labrum (*arrow*) is consistent with a SLAP tear as seen on a coronal oblique FSE T2-weighted fat-saturated sequence. (*B*) MR arthrography confirms the SLAP tear (*arrow*) on a coronal oblique FSE T1-weighted fat-saturated sequence.

The coronal and axial T2-weighted sequences are used to assess the glenoid labrum. The coronal and sagittal T1-weighted sequences are used to assess for marrow abnormalities, muscle atrophy, and impingement.

Wrist

The evaluation of the wrist by MR imaging has been used ubiquitously with varied success, depending on the indications for the examination. Many orthopedic surgeons continue to advocate conventional tricompartmental arthrography of the wrist for optimal evaluation of the wrist ligaments. An in-depth assessment of the efficacy of MR imaging at current field strengths, as it applies to each structure of the wrist, will elucidate the role for 3T systems. An MR image of the wrist at higher field strengths is sure to improve the diagnostic accuracy; it is hoped that this will convince more orthopedic surgeons of the great usefulness of MR imaging in the assessment of wrist ligament pathology.

Triangular fibrocartilage complex

The assessment of the triangular fibrocartilage (TFC) has had varied success at 1.5T, depending on the study performed. Sensitivities ranged from

54% to 92% and specificities ranged from 41% to 91% [105–107]. In a study by Potter and colleagues [108], a dramatic improvement in routine MR imaging of the TFC was achieved with higher resolution images, with a sensitivity of 100% and a specificity of 97%. This shows promise for higher field strength systems in the evaluation of the wrist.

Several studies assessed the advantages of higher resolution imaging specifically, and demonstrated improved diagnostic accuracy, image quality, SNR, and CNR of the TFC and intercarpal ligaments [109–112]. In the study by Yoshioka and colleagues [111], the SNR of the five different components of the TFC complex was evaluated using high-resolution microscopy coils and conventional wrist coils. Kato and colleagues [109] compared the ability of high-resolution and standard resolution images to detect tears of the TFC; the high-resolution images had improved sensitivity and accuracy.

Two studies demonstrated improved image quality on 3T systems specifically [110,112]. Lenk and colleagues [112] showed improved subjective image quality at 3T compared with 1.5T using the same voxel sizes. Saupe and colleagues [110] found that the TFC was more visible on 3T images when compared with 1.5T images using the same resolution. They showed that the SNR of muscle, bone, and

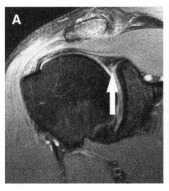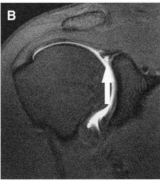

Figure 9 SLAP II tear seen only on MR arthrography. (*A*) Degenerative signal in the superior labrum (*arrow*) prospectively called a possible SLAP I on a coronal oblique FSE T2-weighted fat-saturated sequence from a 3T MR image. (*B*) MR arthrography demonstrates a SLAP II tear (*arrow*) in the same patient on a coronal oblique FSE T1-weighted fat-saturated sequence.

Table 2: **3T MR imaging shoulder protocol**

Parameters	Coronal FSE T2 FS	Coronal FSE T1	Sagittal FSE T1	Sagittal FSE T2 FS	Axial FSE T2 FS
TR (ms)	2825	500	500	2825	3000
TE (ms)	55	10	10	58	50
ETL	12	3	3	12	12
NEX	3	2	1	3	3
BW (kHz)	25	31.25	31.25	25	25
FOV (cm)	14	14	14	14	14
Phase direction	R to L	R to L	A to P	A to P	A to P
Frequency	320	320	320	320	320
Phase	288	288	288	288	256
Slice (mm)	4	4	4	3	4
Gap (mm)	1	1	1	1	0.2
Time	3:12	2:56	1:36	3:12	3:24

Abbreviations: A, anterior; BW, bandwidth; ETL, echo train length; FOV, field-of-view; L, left; NEX, number of excitations; P, posterior; R, right; TE, echo time; TR, repetition time.

cartilage was almost double on 3T systems compared with 1.5T systems. One drawback of that study was the almost doubling of scan times for several of the sequences, a problem that the author's practice has not experienced, as can be shown in the wrist protocol (see Table 2). The author has experienced an excellent demonstration of the normal and abnormal TFC at 3T, and several of his surgeons have been pleased with the image quality and diagnostic assessment (Fig. 10).

Whether the added spatial resolution of 3T will obviate the need for MR arthrography of the wrist is debatable. Many studies demonstrated an improved TFC lesion detection rate with MR arthrography, with sensitivities of 85% to 97% and specificities of 88% to 100% [107,113–115]. Several investigators also showed success with indirect arthrography [105,116,117]. Likewise, the author has seen several examples of TFC tears that were not detected on routine 3T MR images, but that were

discovered after MR arthrography (Fig. 11). Therefore, the higher resolution that is available with 3T systems may decrease the number of necessary arthrograms, but it is not likely to replace them completely.

Scapholunate and lunotriquetral ligaments

The routine MR imaging evaluation of the scapholunate ligament has been disappointing at best, with sensitivities of 11% to 69% and specificities of 34% to 100% [104–107,118,119]. The success rate is even worse when evaluating the lunotriquetral ligament [105–107], with sensitivities of 0% to 36% and specificities of 81% to 99%. Because of the enhanced SNR and spatial resolution, the author has noticed that the intrinsic ligaments of the wrist are seen more easily at 3T (Fig. 12). As a result, he believes that tears of the scapholunate ligament (Fig. 13) and lunotriquetral ligament (Fig. 14) are demonstrated better at 3T.

The diagnostic ability improves with direct arthrography for the scapholunate ligament as shown in several reports; sensitivities reach 56% to 92% with specificities of 52% to 100% [107,113–115,119,120]. Some investigators showed some success with indirect arthrography [105,117,118]. Improving the diagnosis of lunotriquetral ligament tears remains elusive, however; one report showed sensitivities of 23% to 36% and a specificity of 94% [107] with direct arthrography. The author commonly uses MR arthrography for the evaluation of the intrinsic ligaments of the wrist even at 3T, and often is surprised by the change in the diagnosis that was based initially on the routine MR images.

The preliminary data that demonstrated improved visibility and CNR of the scapholunate and lunotriquetral ligaments indicate a promising

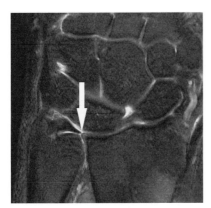

Figure 10 A tear of the TFC (*arrow*) is demonstrated on 3T MR images using a coronal FSE T2-weighted fat-saturated sequence.

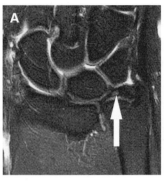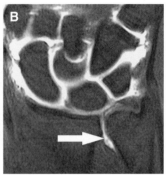

Figure 11 TFC tear is not seen on routine 3T MR images. (*A*) Degenerative signal seen in the TFC (*arrow*) on a coronal FSE T2-weighted fat-saturated image. (*B*) MR arthrography of the same patient demonstrates fluid in the distal radioulnar joint (*arrow*) on a coronal FSE T1-weighted fat-saturated image; this signifies a tear of the TFC.

role for 3T in the evaluation of the intercarpal ligaments [110,112]. In the study by Lenk and colleagues [112], which used similar voxel sizes on a 3T MR image and a 1.5T MR image, the intrinsic ligaments of the wrist had improved visibility at 3T. Likewise, Saupe and colleagues [110] found a subjective increase in the visibility of the scapholunate and lunotriquetral ligaments at 3T compared with 1.5T using similar spatial resolution. These studies bode well for the ability of 3T MR imaging to provide a dramatic improvement in the diagnosis of ligament pathology in the wrist.

How it is done

The author uses the Mayo Clinic (Rochester, Minnesota) single-channel receive-only wrist coil on a GE 3T MR imaging system with the HD Excite platform. Five sequences are acquired for a total scan time of 13 minutes and 2 seconds in a 30-minute time slot. The following five sequences and are used: coronal FSE T2 with fat saturation, coronal FSE T1, sagittal

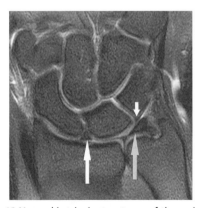

Figure 12 Normal intrinsic structures of the wrist demonstrated on a coronal FSE T2-weighted image with fat saturation obtained at 3T. The scapholunate ligament (*long white arrow*), TFC (*long gray arrow*), and lunotriquetral ligament (*short white arrow*) are shown in excellent detail.

FSE T2 with fat saturation, axial FSE T2 with fat saturation, and axial FSE T1 (Table 3).

The T2-weighed sequences in the coronal plane are used to assess the intrinsic ligaments, extrinsic ligaments, TFC, and marrow abnormalities. The coronal, sagittal, and axial T2-weighted sequences are used to assess the flexor and extensor tendons as well as any soft tissue lesions, such as ganglion cysts. The coronal and axial T1-weighted sequences are used to assess for marrow abnormalities.

Hip

The evaluation of hip pathology by MR imaging has been a successful endeavor. MR imaging is an accurate examination for the assessment of avascular necrosis, transient marrow edema, and insufficiency fractures [121,122]. MR imaging also has been applied in the work-up of patients who have labral or cartilage pathology; however, when evaluating the acetabular labrum and the articular cartilage, MR imaging performs less impressively. This creates the perfect application for higher-field strength systems, such as 3T MR imaging, to improve on current accuracies.

Cartilage

Diagnosing disorders of the articular cartilage of the hip has important implications for older patients who have osteoarthritis and for younger patients who have femoroacetabular impingement [123]. Many investigators demonstrated varied success in the assessment of the articular cartilage of the hip using conventional MR images on current field strength systems [124,125], likely because of the difficulty in visualizing the thin rim of cartilage that overlies the femoral head and acetabulum. Normal acetabular cartilage was reported to be as thin as 1.34 mm [126], and normal femoral cartilage was reported to be as thin as 1.1 mm [127]. One study demonstrated excellent correlation between the radiologist's grading of cartilage pathology and the surgical grading using nonarthrographic MR images [128].

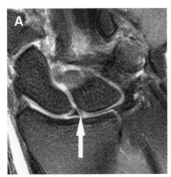
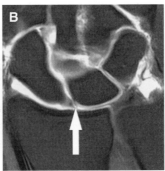

Figure 13 Tear of the scapholunate ligament demonstrated at 3T. (*A*) A coronal FSE T2-weighted fat-saturated image demonstrates fluid within the scapholunate ligament (*arrow*). (*B*) MR arthrogram of the same patient shows contrast filling the tear of the scapholunate ligament (*arrow*) and contrast pooling in the midcarpal joint after radiocarpal injection as seen on a coronal FSE T1-weighted fat-saturated image.

Direct MR arthrography has been advocated to enhance the detection of intra-articular disorders of the hip [129]. Even with the use of direct MR arthrography, the ability to detect cartilage lesions is suboptimal [123,130] as seen in a study by Keeney and colleagues [130] who had a sensitivity of 47% and an accuracy of 67%. Knuesel and colleagues [131] attempted to improve the cartilage lesion visibility on postarthrographic MR images by comparing a 3D water-excitation technique with standard T1-weighted spin-echo images. Although the articular cartilage appeared more visible, the diagnostic accuracy was not improved, with a sensitivity of detection as low as 58%.

The assessment of the articular cartilage of the hip is well suited for 3T MR imaging, because of the gain in signal and spatial resolution that are needed to evaluate such a small structure relative to the other structures of the hip. Rubin and colleagues [132] found that higher resolution imaging at 1.5T improved the visibility of hip cartilage. Anecdotally, the author has experienced subjective improvement in the appearance of the cartilage of the femoral head and acetabular fossa with 3T (Fig. 15).

Labrum

Pathologic conditions of the acetabular labrum may be seen in patients who have femoracetabaular impingement [133,134], developmental dysplasia of the hip [134], or osteoarthritis [134] as well as in athletes [135] and patients who have sustained trauma [136]. Therefore, the diagnosis of labral tears is an important goal for MR imaging; however, routine MR has not satisfactorily met diagnostic expectations. Several reports elucidated the disappointing results of routine MR imaging in the evaluation of labral disease, with a sensitivity of approximately 65% [137]. One study, however, achieved excellent correlation between MR imaging findings and arthroscopy [128]. In the author's practice, the acetabular labrum has been more visible on 3T imaging and it has become easier to detect labral pathology (Fig. 16).

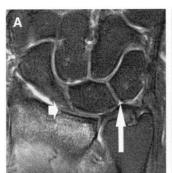
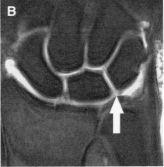

Figure 14 Tear of the lunotriquetral ligament demonstrated at 3T. (*A*) A coronal FSE T2-weighted fat-saturated image shows fluid in the expected location of the lunotriquetral ligament (*long arrow*). An incidental distal radial fracture is demonstrated extending to the articular surface (*short arrow*). (*B*) MR arthrogram in the same patient shows contrast filling the lunotriquetral ligament (*arrow*) and extending into the midcarpal joint after radiocarpal injection as seen on a coronal FSE T1-weighted fat-saturated image.

Table 3: **3T MR imaging wrist protocol**

Parameters	Coronal FSE T2 FS	Coronal FSE T1	Sagittal FSE T2 FS	Axial FSE T2 FS	Axial FSE T1
TR (ms)	4050	450	3100	3100	500
TE (ms)	55	11	55	55	16
ETL	12	3	12	12	3
NEX	2	1	2	2	1
BW (kHz)	25	31.25	25	25	31.25
FOV (cm)	10	10	10	10	10
Phase direction	S to I	S to I	S to I	R to L	R to L
Frequency	384	384	384	384	384
Phase	288	320	288	288	320
Slice (mm)	3	3	3	3	3
Gap (mm)	0	0	1	1	1
Time	3:19	2:37	2:35	2:35	1:56

The parameters are optimized for the GE 3T MR imaging system with the HD Excite platform.
Abbreviations: BW, bandwidth; ETL, echo train length; FOV, field-of-view; I, inferior; L, left; NEX, number of excitations; R, right; S, superior; TE, echo time; TR, repetition time.

Direct MR arthrography has proven to be superior to routine MR imaging in demonstrating tears of the labrum [122,134,137–139]; the literature reports a sensitivity of between 92% and 95% [137]. Rubin and colleagues [132] showed that high-resolution images can elucidate the labrum in better detail with improved visibility. This lends evidence to a well-suited role for the high spatial resolution that is afforded by 3T MR imaging in the assessment of the acetabular labrum.

How it is done

The author uses the USA Instruments eight-channel, phased-array, receive-only torso coil for routine hip imaging on a GE 3T MR imaging system with an HD Excite platform. Six sequences are used: large FOV coronal FSE T2 with fat saturation using a parallel imaging acceleration factor of 2 (ASSET [array spatial sensitivity encoding technique]), large FOV coronal FSE T1 with a parallel imaging acceleration factor of 2 (ASSET), small FOV coronal FSE T2 with fat saturation, small FOV coronal FSE T1, sagittal FSE T2 with fat saturation, and axial FSE T1 (Table 4). The total scan time, excluding patient set-up and prescanning, is 23 minutes and 2 seconds. Patients are scheduled into 30-minute time slots. Parallel imaging is not suited for the small FOV images because of the vulnerability to wrap-around artifact. For optimal use of parallel imaging, the entire anatomy must be included in the phase FOV.

The author's large FOV sequences allow for comparison of the signal in the contralateral hip, as well as the identification of other pain sources that can occur throughout the pelvis, such as stress fractures. In addition, because avascular necrosis (AVN) of the hip often is bilateral, a large FOV sequence enables the determination of the bilaterality of the disease. The T2-weighted sequences with fat saturation

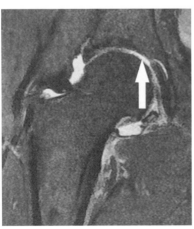

Figure 15 Cartilage loss along the femoral head (*arrow*) is well demonstrated at 3T as seen on a coronal FSE T2-weighted fat-saturated image.

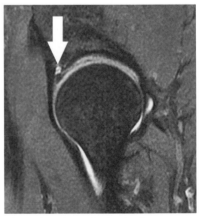

Figure 16 Paralabral cyst (*arrow*) adjacent to the anterosuperior acetabular labrum signifies a tear as seen on a sagittal FSE T2-weighted fat-saturated image obtained at 3T.

Table 4: **3T MR imaging hip protocol**

Parameters	Large FOV coronal FSE T2 FS	Large FOV coronal FSE T1	Small FOV coronal FSE T2 FS	Small FOV coronal FSE T1	Sagittal FSE T2 FS	Small FOV axial FSE T2 FS
TR (ms)	3900	500	4700	500	4450	4450
TE (ms)	55	12	55	10	55	55
ETL	12	3	12	3	12	12
NEX	2	2	3	3	3	3
FOV (cm)	40	40	20	20	20	20
BW (kHz)	25	31.25	25	31.25	25	25
Frequency	512	512	384	320	384	384
Phase	256	256	256	256	256	256
Slice (mm)	6	6	4	4	4	4
Gap (mm)	1	1	1	1	1	1
ASSET	2	2	None	None	None	None
Time	1:57	1:32	5:15	4:22	4:58	4:58

The parameters are optimized for the GE 3T MR imaging system with the HD Excite platform.
Parallel imaging (ASSET) with an acceleration factor of 2 is used on the large FOV sequences.
Abbreviations: ASSET, array spatial sensitivity encoding technique; BW, bandwidth; ETL, echo train length; FOV, field-of-view; NEX, number of excitations; TE, echo time; TR, repetition time.

are used predominantly to assess for marrow abnormalities, bursitis, joint effusions, labral tears, and paralabral cysts. The T1-weighted sequences are excellent for determining the presence of fractures or other marrow lesions as well as any intra-articular bodies. Muscle atrophy or muscle masses also can be assessed on T1-weighted sequences.

Elbow

MR imaging is extremely helpful in the assessment of the osseous structures, tendons, and ligaments of the elbow [140–142]; however, there is much room for improvement in the evaluation of the collateral ligaments.

Collateral ligaments

Timmerman and colleagues [143] demonstrated a dismal sensitivity of 57% and a specificity of 100% in the evaluation of the ulnar collateral ligament by routine MR imaging. By using MR arthrography, one may improve on the accuracy of routine MR images [144–146]. High-resolution MR imaging demonstrated improved visibility of the elbow ligaments [147–149]. In one report, Carrino and colleagues [147] demonstrated optimal evaluation of the lateral ulnar collateral ligament using MR arthrography and high-resolution intermediate-weighted FSE sequences. In another study, Carrino and colleagues [148] showed similar conclusions in the assessment of the ulnar collateral ligament. These findings show promise for the usefulness of 3T imaging in the evaluation of the ligaments of the elbow, with improved spatial resolution and signal. Overall, the author has found that using

3T MR imaging in the elbow has made the evaluation of the collateral ligaments much more efficacious (Fig. 17). His practice continues to rely on MR arthrography for complete assessment of the elbow collateral ligaments, especially in high-performance athletes, because in many cases, the diagnosis has been changed based on the postarthrographic images (Fig. 18).

How it is done

The author uses the MRI Devices eight-channel, phased-array, transmit-receive knee coil or the Medical Advances quadrature, transmit-receive knee coil for elbow imaging on a GE 3T MR imaging system

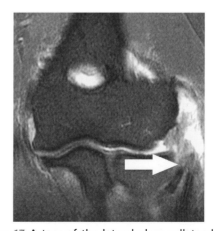

Figure 17 A tear of the lateral ulnar collateral ligament is well demonstrated on 3T MR imaging as seen on a coronal FSE T2-weighted fat-saturated image. The torn tendon (*arrow*) is retracted to the level of the radial head.

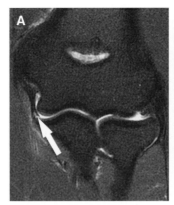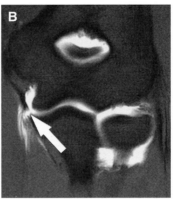

Figure 18 MR arthrography at 3T in a baseball player who complained of medial elbow pain. (*A*) Fluid (*arrow*) at the attachment of the anterior bundle of the ulnar collateral ligament to the sublime tubercle was called a partial tear prospectively as seen on a coronal FSE T2-weighted fat-saturated image. (*B*) MR arthrography in the same patient demonstrates contrast extending through a full-thickness defect (*arrow*) in the anterior bundle into the extracapsular soft tissues as seen on a coronal FSE T1-weighted fat-saturated image.

with the HD Excite platform. Five sequences are acquired for a total scan time of 16 minutes and 39 seconds in a 30-minute time slot. The following sequences are used: coronal FSE T2 with fat saturation, coronal FSE T1, sagittal FSE T2 with fat saturation, axial FSE T1, and axial FSE T2 with fat saturation (Table 5).

The T2-weighed sequences in the coronal plane are used to assess the collateral ligaments. The coronal, sagittal, and axial T2-weighted sequences are used to assess the tendons. The coronal and axial T1-weighted sequences are used to assess for marrow abnormalities, such as fractures and tumors, and for osteochondral lesions and intra-articular bodies. Many investigators advocate the use of gradient echo sequences to assess the collateral ligaments; however, these sequences often are suboptimal for marrow, ligamentous, and tendinous

edema. Therefore, the T2-weighted sequences are optimized to encompass ligament assessment and to detect pathologic edema.

Ankle

The assessment of the many osseous and soft tissue structures of the ankle can be done on routine MR imaging. Deficiencies arise in the evaluation of specific ligamentous structures, however.

Collateral ligaments

The many ligamentous structures of the ankle are demonstrated well on MR imaging [150–156], including the lateral, medial, syndesmotic, and sinus tarsi ligaments. Various success rates in the evaluation of these ligaments have been shown. A sensitivity of 74% and a specificity of 100% were obtained

Table 5: **3T MR imaging elbow protocol**

Parameters	Coronal FSE T2 FS	Coronal FSE T1	Sagittal FSE T2 FS	Axial FSE T2 FS	Axial FSE T1
TR (ms)	3300	625	3300	4300	550
TE (ms)	55	14	55	55	9
ETL	12	3	12	12	3
NEX	3	1	2	2	1
FOV (cm)	14	14	14	14	14
BW (kHz)	25	31.25	25	25	31.25
Phase direction	S to I	S to I	S to I	R to L	R to L
Frequency	384	512	384	384	512
Phase	320	320	320	320	320
Slice (mm)	3	3	3	3	3
Gap (mm)	0	0	1	1	1
Time	4:34	2:00	3:16	4:00	2:49

Abbreviations: BW, bandwidth; ETL, echo train length; FOV, field-of-view; I, inferior; L, left; NEX, number of excitations; R, right; S, superior; TE, echo time; TR, repetition time.

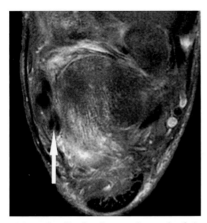

Figure 19 Longitudinal split tear (*arrow*) of the calcaneofibular ligament is demonstrated well on an axial FSE T2-weighted fat-saturated image obtained on a 3T MR imaging scanner.

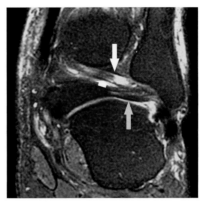

Figure 20 Posterior ankle ligaments are demonstrated well on a coronal FSE T2-weighted fat-saturated image obtained a 3T MR imaging system. The transverse ligament (*long white arrow*), the intermalleolar ligament or tibial slip (*short white arrow*), and the posterior talofibular ligament (*long gray arrow*) are seen well.

for the entire lateral complex [157]. For the anterior talofibular ligament, sensitivities of 100% and specificities of 50% to 100% were shown [158,159]. For the posterior talofibular ligament, a sensitivity of 33% and a specificity of 78% were demonstrated [159]. For the calcaneofibular ligament, sensitivities of 64% to 92% and specificities of 100% were shown [158,159]. The accuracy of MR imaging in the assessment of deltoid ligament tears has not been investigated fully. Clearly, there is a role for 3T MR imaging in improving the detection of pathology that involves the posterior talofibular ligament and the calcaneofibular ligament. Muhle and colleagues [160] demonstrated that high-resolution images with an 8-cm FOV, 3-mm slice thickness, and a 256 × 256 matrix that were obtained on a 1.5T system were capable of displaying the lateral

and medial ligaments with perfect anatomic resolution as compared with cadaveric correlation. The author has found excellent demonstration of these ligaments on his 3T system, and diagnoses tears more confidently (Fig. 19).

Syndesmotic ligamentous complex

Excellent results also have been demonstrated for the evaluation of the syndesmotic complex, with sensitivities of 100% for the anterior and posterior tibiofibular ligaments [161,162]. A study by Muhle and colleagues [163] attempted to show the benefits of high-resolution images of the ankle using a specialized local coil in demonstrating the syndesmotic ligaments. They found that there was excellent correlation in the appearance of the

Table 6: 3T MR imaging ankle protocol					
Parameters	Sagittal FSE T2 FS	Sagittal FSE T1	Axial FSE PD	Axial FSE T2 FS	Coronal FSE T2 FS
TR (ms)	2850	500	2450	3950	4350
TE (ms)	55	10	13	55	55
ETL	12	3	5	12	12
NEX	3	1	1	2	2
FOV (cm)	16	16	15	15	15
BW (kHz)	25	31.25	31.25	25	25
Phase direction	S to I	S to I	R to L	R to L	S to I
Frequency	384	384	512	320	320
Phase	320	320	384	320	320
Slice (mm)	4	4	4	4	4
Gap (mm)	1	1	0.5	0.5	1
Time	3:57	1:56	3:16	3:49	4:08

The parameters are optimized for the GE 3T MR imaging system with the HD Excite platform.
Abbreviations: BW, bandwidth; ETL, echo train length; FOV, field-of-view; I, inferior; L, left; NEX, number of excitations; R, right; S, superior; TE, echo time; TR, repetition time.

ligaments and cadaveric anatomic sections. This lends support to the concept that the additional field strength, spatial resolution, and SNR that are afforded by 3T systems will serve as an excellent tool in the evaluation of syndesmotic ligament pathology. In keeping with this, the author has been able to demonstrate the normal structures of the syndesmotic ligamentous complex beautifully with 3T (Fig. 20) and to diagnose tears.

How it is done

The author uses the Medical Advances quadrature transmit-receive knee coil with chimney component, which allows for neutral ankle positioning, on a GE 3T MR imaging system with the HD Excite platform. Five sequences are acquired for a total scan time of 17 minutes and 6 seconds in a 30-minute time slot. The following sequences are used: sagittal FSE T2 with fat saturation, sagittal FSE T1, axial FSE PD, axial FSE T2 with fat saturation, and coronal FSE T2 with fat saturation (Table 6).

The T2 and PD-weighted sequences are used to assess the ligaments, tendons, and cartilage. The sagittal T1-weighted sequences are used to assess for marrow abnormalities.

Summary

The gain in SNR that is afforded by 3T MR imaging systems has tremendous clinical applications in the musculoskeletal system. The potential for demonstrating and enhancing the visibility of normal osseous, tendinous, cartilaginous, and ligamentous structures is exciting. Furthermore, harnessing this added signal to increase spatial resolution may improve our diagnostic abilities in various joints dramatically. Radiologists have enjoyed great success in assessing joint disease with current MR imaging field strengths; however, many intrinsic joint structures remain poorly evaluated, which leads to a golden opportunity for 3T MR imaging. The articular cartilage of the knee, the glenoid labrum of the shoulder, the intrinsic ligaments and TFC of the wrist, the collateral ligaments of the elbow, the labrum and articular cartilage of the hip, and the collateral ligaments of the ankle have been evaluated suboptimally on 1.5T systems using routine nonarthrographic MR images.

Because of the enhanced SNR, the higher spatial resolution, and the greater CNR of intrinsic joint structures at higher field strengths, 3T MR imaging has the potential to improve diagnostic abilities in the musculoskeletal system vastly, which translates into better patient care and management. The author's 2 years of clinical experience with musculoskeletal MR imaging on 3T systems has met and exceeded his expectations, and has bolstered the confidence of his orthopedic surgeons in his diagnoses. As coil technology advances and as the use of parallel imaging becomes more available in the extremities, the author expects to see even more dramatic improvements in image quality.

References

[1] Jee WH, McCauley TR, Kim JM. Magnetic resonance diagnosis of meniscal tears in patients with acute anterior cruciate ligament tears. J Comput Assist Tomogr 2004;28:402–6.

[2] Dorsey TA, Helms CA. Bucket-handle meniscal tears of the knee: sensitivity and specificity of MRI signs. Skeletal Radiol 2003;32:266–72.

[3] Munshi M, Davidson M, MacDonald PB, et al. The efficacy of magnetic resonance imaging in acute knee injuries. Clin J Sport Med 2000; 10:34–9.

[4] Cheung LP, Li KC, Hollett MD, et al. Meniscal tears of the knee: accuracy of detection with fast spin-echo MR imaging and arthroscopic correlation in 293 patients. Radiology 1997; 203(2):508–12.

[5] Muellner T, Weinstabl R, Schabus R, et al. The diagnosis of meniscal tears in athletes. A comparison of clinical and magnetic resonance imaging investigations. Am J Sports Med 1997; 25:7–12.

[6] Escobedo EM, Hunter JC, Zink-Brody GC, et al. Usefulness of turbo spin-echo MR imaging in the evaluation of meniscal tears: comparison with a conventional spin-echo sequence. AJR Am J Roentgenol 1996;167:1223–7.

[7] Magee TH, Hinson GW. MRI of meniscal bucket-handle tears. Skeletal Radiol 1998;27:495–9.

[8] Elvenes J, Jerome CP, Reikeras O, et al. Magnetic resonance imaging as a screening procedure to avoid arthroscopy for meniscal tears. Arch Orthop Trauma Surg 2000;120:14–6.

[9] Feller JA, Webster KE. Clinical value of magnetic resonance imaging of the knee. ANZ J Surg 2001;71:534–7.

[10] Rose NE, Gold SM. A comparison of accuracy between clinical examination and magnetic resonance imaging in the diagnosis of meniscal and anterior cruciate ligament tears. Arthroscopy 1996;12:398–405.

[11] Ghanem I, Abou Jaoude S, Kharrat K, et al. Is MRI effective in detecting intraarticular abnormalities of the injured knee? J Med Liban 2002;50:168–74.

[12] Kocabey Y, Tetik O, Isbell WM, et al. The value of clinical examination versus magnetic resonance imaging in the diagnosis of meniscal tears and anterior cruciate ligament rupture. Arthroscopy 2004;20:696–700.

[13] Stanitski CL. Correlation of arthroscopic and clinical examinations with magnetic resonance imaging findings of injured knees in children and adolescents. Am J Sports Med 1998;26:2–6.

[14] Bugnone AN, Ramnath RR, Davis SB, et al. The quadruple cruciate sign of simultaneous bicompartmental medial and lateral bucket-handle meniscal tears. Skeletal Radiol 2005;34(11): 740–4.

[15] Ha TP, Li KC, Beaulieu CF, et al. Anterior cruciate ligament injury: fast spin-echo MR imaging with arthroscopic correlation in 217 examinations. AJR Am J Roentgenol 1998;170: 1215–9.

[16] Vellet AD, Lee DH, Munk PL, et al. Anterior cruciate ligament tear: prospective evaluation of diagnostic accuracy of middle- and high-field-strength MR imaging at 1.5 and 0.5T. Radiology 1995;197:826–30.

[17] Barry KP, Mesgarzadeh M, Triolo J, et al. Accuracy of MRI patterns in evaluating anterior cruciate ligament tears. Skeletal Radiol 1996; 25:365–70.

[18] Friedman RL, Jackson DW. Magnetic resonance imaging of the anterior cruciate ligament: current concepts. Orthopedics 1996;19:525–32.

[19] Munk PL, Hilborn MD, Vellet AD, et al. Diagnostic equivalence of conventional and fast spin echo magnetic resonance imaging of the anterior cruciate ligament of the knee. Australas Radiol 1997;41:238–42.

[20] Sasaki T, Saito Y, Yodono H, et al. MR diagnosis of internal derangement of the knee by SE T1 and GRE T2* weighted images: evaluation of 300 arthroscopically proven knees. Nippon Igaku Hoshasen Gakkai Zasshi 1998;58:572–7.

[21] Mellado JM, Calmet J, Olona M, et al. Magnetic resonance imaging of the anterior cruciate ligament tears: reevaluation of quantitative parameters and imaging findings including a simplified method for measuring the anterior cruciate ligament angle. Knee Surg Sports Traumatol Arthrosc 2004;12:217–24.

[22] Umans H, Wimpfheimer O, Haramati N, et al. Diagnosis of partial tears of the anterior cruciate ligament of the knee: value of MR imaging. AJR Am J Roentgenol 1995;165:893–7.

[23] Moore SL. Imaging the anterior cruciate ligament. Orthop Clin North Am 2002;33:663–74.

[24] Servant CT, Ramos JP, Thomas NP. The accuracy of magnetic resonance imaging in diagnosing chronic posterior cruciate ligament injury. Knee 2004;11:265–70.

[25] Vahey TN, Broome DR, Kayes KJ, et al. Acute and chronic tears of the anterior cruciate ligament: differential features at MR imaging. Radiology 1991;181:251–3.

[26] Yao L, Gentili A, Petrus L, et al. Partial ACL rupture: an MR diagnosis? Skeletal Radiol 1995; 24:247–51.

[27] Gross ML, Grover JS, Bassett LW, et al. Magnetic resonance imaging of the posterior cruciate ligament. Clinical use to improve diagnostic accuracy. Am J Sports Med 1992;20:732–7.

[28] Chen MC, Shih TT, Jiang CC, et al. MRI of meniscus and cruciate ligament tears correlated with arthroscopy. J Formos Med Assoc 1995; 94:605–11.

[29] Hodler J, Buess E, Rodriguez M, et al. Magnetic resonance tomography of the knee joint: meniscus, cruciate ligaments, and hyaline cartilage. Rofo 1993;159:107–12.

[30] Vallotton JA, Meuli RA, Leyvraz PF, et al. Comparison between magnetic resonance imaging and arthroscopy in the diagnosis of patellar cartilage lesions: a prospective study. Knee Surg Sports Traumatol Arthrosc 1995;3:157–62.

[31] Suh JS, Cho JH, Shin KH, et al. Chondromalacia of the knee: evaluation with a fat-suppression three-dimensional SPGR imaging after intravenous contrast injection. J Magn Reson Imaging 1996;6:884–8.

[32] Potter HG, Linklater JM, Allen AA, et al. Magnetic resonance imaging of articular cartilage in the knee. An evaluation with use of fast-spin-echo imaging. J Bone Joint Surg Am 1998; 80:1276–84.

[33] Kreitner KF, Hansen M, Schadmand-Fischer S, et al. Low-field MRI of the knee joint: results of a prospective, arthroscopically controlled study. Rofo 1999;170:35–40.

[34] Bredella MA, Tirman PF, Peterfy CG, et al. Accuracy of T2-weighted fast spin-echo MR imaging with fat saturation in detecting cartilage defects in the knee: comparison with arthroscopy in 130 patients. AJR Am J Roentgenol 1999; 172:1073–80.

[35] Sonin AH, Pensy RA, Mulligan ME, et al. Grading articular cartilage of the knee using fast spin-echo proton density-weighted MR imaging without fat suppression. AJR Am J Roentgenol 2002;179:1159–66.

[36] Friemert B, Oberlander Y, Danz B, et al. MRI vs. arthroscopy in the diagnosis of cartilage lesions in the knee. Can MRI take place of arthroscopy? Zentralbl Chir 2002;127:822–7.

[37] Mohr A. The value of water-excitation 3D FLASH and fat-saturated PDw TSE MR imaging for detecting and grading articular cartilage lesions of the knee. Skeletal Radiol 2003;32:396–402.

[38] Macarini L, Perrone A, Murrone M, et al. Evaluation of patellar chondromalacia with MR: comparison between T2-weighted FSE SPIR and GE MTC. Radiol Med (Torino) 2004;108:159–71.

[39] Ruehm S, Zanetti M, Romero J, et al. MRI of patellar articular cartilage: evaluation of an optimized gradient echo sequence (3D-DESS). J Magn Reson Imaging 1998;8:1246–51.

[40] Lee SH, Suh JS, Cho J, et al. Evaluation of chondromalacia of the patella with axial inversion recovery-fast spin-echo imaging. J Magn Reson Imaging 2001;13:412–6.

[41] Murphy BJ. Evaluation of grades 3 and 4 chondromalacia of the knee using T2*-weighted 3D gradient-echo articular cartilage imaging. Skeletal Radiol 2001;30:305–11.

[42] Macarini L, Murrone M, Marini S, et al. MR in the study of knee cartilage pathologies:

influence of location and grade on the effectiveness of the method. Radiol Med (Torino) 2003; 105:296–307.

[43] Rubenstein JD, Li JG, Majumdar S, et al. Image resolution and signal-to-noise ratio requirements for MR imaging of degenerative cartilage. AJR Am J Roentgenol 1997;169:1089–96.

[44] Gold GE, Han E, Stainsby J, et al. Musculoskeletal MRI at 3.0T: relaxation times and image contrast. AJR Am J Roentgenol 2004;183:343–51.

[45] Schroder RJ, Fischbach F, Unterhauser FN, et al. Value of various MR sequences using 1.5 and 3.0 Tesla in analyzing cartilaginous defects of the patella in an animal model. Rofo 2004; 176:1667–75.

[46] Fischbach F, Bruhn H, Unterhauser F, et al. Magnetic resonance imaging of hyaline cartilage defects at 1.5T and 3.0T: comparison of medium T2-weighted fast spin echo, T1-weighted two-dimensional and three-dimensional gradient echo pulse sequences. Acta Radiol 2005; 46:67–73.

[47] Kendell SD, Helms CA, Rampton JW, et al. MRI appearance of chondral delamination injuries of the knee. AJR Am J Roentgenol 2005; 184:1486–9.

[48] Mosher TJ, Dardzinski BJ, Smith MB. Human articular cartilage: influence of aging and early symptomatic degeneration on the spatial variation of T2-preliminary findings at 3T. Radiology 2000;214:259–66.

[49] Mosher TJ, Dardzinski BJ. Cartilage MRI T2 relaxation time mapping: overview and applications. Semin Musculoskelet Radiol 2004; 8:355–68.

[50] Dunn TC, Lu Y, Jin H, et al. T2 relaxation time of cartilage at MR imaging: comparison with severity of knee osteoarthritis. Radiology 2004; 232:592–8.

[51] Watrin-Pinzano A, Ruaud JP, Olivier P, et al. Effect of proteoglycan depletion on T2 mapping in rat patellar cartilage. Radiology 2005;234: 162–70.

[52] Watrin A, Ruaud JP, Olivier PTA, et al. T2 mapping of rat patellar cartilage. Radiology 2001; 219:395–402.

[53] Loeuille D, Olivier P, Watrin A, et al. The biochemical content of articular cartilage: an original MRI approach. Biorheology 2002;39:269–76.

[54] Goodwin DW, Wadghiri YZ, Zhu H, et al. Macroscopic structure of articular cartilage of the tibial plateau: influence of a characteristic matrix architecture on MRI appearance. AJR Am J Roentgenol 2004;182:311–8.

[55] Breuseghem IV, Bosmans HTC, Elst LV, et al. T2 mapping of human femorotibial cartilage with turbo mixed MR imaging at 1.5T: feasibility. Radiology 2004;233:609–14.

[56] Dardzinski BJ, Laor T, Schmithorst VJ, et al. Mapping T2 relaxation time in the pediatric knee: feasibility with a clinical 1.5T MR imaging system. Radiology 2002;225:233–9.

[57] Tardieu M, Lazennec JY, Christel P, et al. Normal and pathological MRI aspects of the posterolateral corner of the knee. J Radiol 1995; 76:605–9.

[58] Verma NN, Mithofer K, Battaglia M, et al. The docking technique for posterolateral corner reconstruction. Arthroscopy 2005;21: 238–42.

[59] Stannard JP, Brown SL, Farris RC, et al. The posterolateral corner of the knee. Am J Sports Med 2005;33(6):881–8. Epub 2005 Apr 12.

[60] Kocabey Y, Nawab A, Caborn DN, et al. Posterolateral corner reconstruction using a hamstring allograft and a bioabsorbable tenodesis screw: description of a new surgical technique. Arthroscopy 2004;20:159–63.

[61] Kimori K, Suzu F, Yamashita F, et al. Evaluation of arthrography and arthroscopy for lesions of the posteromedial corner of the knee. Am J Sports Med 1989;17:638–43.

[62] Sims WF, Jacobson KE. The posteromedial corner of the knee: medial-sided injury patterns revisited. Am J Sports Med 2004;32:337–45.

[63] Robinson JR, Sanchez-Ballester J, Bull AMJ, et al. The posteromedial corner revisited: an anatomical description of the passive restraining structures of the medial aspect of the human knee. J Bone Joint Surg Br 2004;86B:674–81.

[64] Iannotti JP, Zlatkin MB, Esterhai JL, et al. Magnetic resonance imaging of the shoulder. Sensitivity, specificity, and predictive value. J Bone Joint Surg Am 1991;73:17–29.

[65] Vahlensieck M, Sommer T. Indirect MR arthrography of the shoulder. An alternative to direct MR arthrography? Radiologe 1996;36:960–5.

[66] Zhu Q, Katsuya N. Normal anatomy and related pathological changes of shoulder on MRI. Zhonghua Wai Ke Za Zhi 2000;38:259–62.

[67] Yamakawa S, Hashizume H, Ichikawa N, et al. Comparative studies of MRI and operative findings in rotator cuff tear. Acta Med Okayama 2001;55:261–8.

[68] Tuite MJ, Asinger D, Orwin JF. Angled oblique sagittal MR imaging of rotator cuff tears: comparison with standard oblique sagittal images. Skeletal Radiol 2001;30:262–9.

[69] Kenn W, Hufnagel P, Muller T, et al. Arthrography, ultrasound and MRI in rotator cuff lesions: a comparison of methods in partial lesions and small complete ruptures. Rofo 2000;172: 260–6.

[70] Blanchard TK, Bearcroft PW, Constant CR, et al. Diagnostic and therapeutic impact of MRI and arthrography in the investigation of full-thickness rotator cuff tears. Eur Radiol 1999;9: 638–42.

[71] Sahin-Akyar G, Miller TT, Staron RB, et al. Gradient-echo versus fat-suppressed fast spin-echo MR imaging of rotator cuff tears. AJR Am J Roentgenol 1998;171:223–7.

[72] Low R, Kreitner KF, Runkel M, et al. Low-field MR arthrography of the shoulder: early results

using an open 0.2T MR system. Rofo 1998; 168:316–22.

[73] Wnorowski DC, Levinsohn EM, Chamberlain BC, et al. Magnetic resonance imaging assessment of the rotator cuff: is it really accurate? Arthroscopy 1997;13:710–9.

[74] Balich SM, Sheley RC, Brown TR, et al. MR imaging of the rotator cuff tendon: interobserver agreement and analysis of interpretive errors. Radiology 1997;204:191–4.

[75] Sonin AH, Peduto AJ, Fitzgerald SW, et al. MR imaging of the rotator cuff mechanism: comparison of spin-echo and turbo spin-echo sequences. AJR Am J Roentgenol 1996;167: 333–8.

[76] Reinus WR, Shady KL, Mirowitz SA, et al. MR diagnosis of rotator cuff tears of the shoulder: value of using T2-weighted fat-saturated images. AJR Am J Roentgenol 1995;164:1451–5.

[77] Robertson PL, Schweitzer ME, Mitchell DG, et al. Rotator cuff disorders: interobserver and intraobserver variation in diagnosis with MR imaging. Radiology 1995;194:831–5.

[78] Evancho AM, Stiles RG, Fajman WA, et al. MR imaging diagnosis of rotator cuff tears. AJR Am J Roentgenol 1988;151:751–4.

[79] Guo A, Fujita K, Mizuno K. Diagnostic value of arthrography and MRI in rotator cuff tears. Zhonghua Wai Ke Za Zhi 2000;38:263–5.

[80] Schroder RJ, Bostanjoglo M, Kaab M, et al. Accuracy of routine MRI in lesions of the supraspinatus tendon—comparison with surgical findings. Rofo 2003;175:920–8.

[81] Teefey SA, Rubin DA, Middleton WD, et al. Detection and quantification of rotator cuff tears. Comparison of ultrasonographic, magnetic resonance imaging, and arthroscopic findings in seventy-one consecutive cases. J Bone Joint Surg Am 2004;86-A:708–16.

[82] Palmer WE, Brown JH, Rosenthal DI. Rotator cuff: evaluation with fat-suppressed MR arthrography. Radiology 1993;188:683–7.

[83] Parmar H, Jhankaria B, Maheshwari M, et al. Magnetic resonance arthrography in recurrent anterior shoulder instability as compared to arthroscopy: a prospective comparative study. J Postgrad Med 2002;48:270–3.

[84] Meister K, Thesing J, Montgomery WJ, et al. MR arthrography of partial thickness tears of the undersurface of the rotator cuff: an arthroscopic correlation. Skeletal Radiol 2004;33:136–41.

[85] Green MR, Christensen KP. Magnetic resonance imaging of the glenoid labrum in anterior shoulder instability. Am J Sports Med 1994; 22:493–8.

[86] Tuite MJ, De Smet AA, Norris MA, et al. Anteroinferior tears of the glenoid labrum: fat-suppressed fast spin-echo T2 versus gradient-recalled echo MR images. Skeletal Radiol 1997; 26:293–7.

[87] Tuite MJ, Shinners TJ, Hollister MC, et al. Fat-suppressed fast spin-echo mid-TE (TE (effective) = 34) MR images: comparison with fast spin-echo T2-weighted images for the diagnosis of tears and anatomic variants of the glenoid labrum. Skeletal Radiol 1999; 28:685–90.

[88] Tuite MJ, De Smet AA, Norris MA, et al. MR diagnosis of labral tears of the shoulder: value of T2*-weighted gradient-recalled echo images made in external rotation. AJR Am J Roentgenol 1995;164:941–4.

[89] Yoneda M, Izawa K, Hirooka A, et al. Indicators of superior glenoid labral detachment on magnetic resonance imaging and computed tomography arthrography. J Shoulder Elbow Surg 1998;7:2–12.

[90] Tuite MJ, Cirillo RL, De Smet AA, et al. Superior labrum anterior-posterior (SLAP) tears: evaluation of three MR signs on T2-weighted images. Radiology 2000;215:841–5.

[91] Liu SH, Henry MH, Nuccion S, et al. Diagnosis of glenoid labral tears. A comparison between magnetic resonance imaging and clinical examinations. Am J Sports Med 1996;24:149–54.

[92] Stetson WB, Templin K. The crank test, the O'Brien test, and routine magnetic resonance imaging scans in the diagnosis of labral tears. Am J Sports Med 2002;30:806–9.

[93] Connell DA, Potter HG, Wickiewicz TL, et al. Noncontrast magnetic resonance imaging of superior labral lesions. 102 cases confirmed at arthroscopic surgery. Am J Sports Med 1999; 27:208–13.

[94] Drescher R, Rothenburg TV, Ludwig J, et al. Direct MR-arthrography of the shoulder with maximum capsular distension for surgical planning. Rofo 2004;176:1469–74.

[95] Applegate GR, Hewitt M, Snyder SJ, et al. Chronic labral tears: value of magnetic resonance arthrography in evaluating the glenoid labrum and labral-bicipital complex. Arthroscopy 2004;20:959–63.

[96] Bencardino JT, Beltran J, Rosenberg ZS, et al. Superior labrum anterior-posterior lesions: diagnosis with MR arthrography of the shoulder. Radiology 2000;214:267–71.

[97] Palmer WE, Caslowitz PL. Anterior shoulder instability: diagnostic criteria determined from prospective analysis of 121 MR arthrograms. Radiology 1995;197:819–25.

[98] Wulker N, Ruhmann O. MRI in dislocation and instability of the shoulder joint. Orthopade 2001;30:492–501.

[99] Jee WH, McCauley TR, Katz LD, et al. Superior labral anterior posterior (SLAP) lesions of the glenoid labrum: reliability and accuracy of MR arthrography for diagnosis. Radiology 2001; 218:127–32.

[100] Cvitanic O, Tirman PF, Feller JF, et al. Using abduction and external rotation of the shoulder to increase the sensitivity of MR arthrography in revealing tears of the anterior glenoid labrum. AJR Am J Roentgenol 1997;169:837–44.

[101] Wagner SC, Schweitzer ME, Morrison WB, et al. Shoulder instability: accuracy of MR imaging performed after surgery in depicting recurrent injury—initial findings. Radiology 2002; 222:196–203.

[102] Herold T, Hente R, Zorger N, et al. Indirect MR-arthrography of the shoulder-value in the detection of SLAP-lesions. Rofo 2003;175: 1508–14.

[103] Tung GA, Entzian D, Green A, et al. High-field and low-field MR imaging of superior glenoid labral tears and associated tendon injuries. AJR Am J Roentgenol 2000;174:1107–14.

[104] Magee TM, Shapiro M, Williams D. Comparison of high-field-strength versus low-field-strength MRI of the shoulder. AJR Am J Roentgenol 2003;181:1211–5.

[105] Haims AH, Schweitzer ME, Morrison WB, et al. Internal derangement of the wrist: indirect MR arthrography versus unenhanced MR imaging. Radiology 2003;227:701–7.

[106] Johnstone DJ, Thorogood S, Smith WH, et al. A comparison of magnetic resonance imaging and arthroscopy in the investigation of chronic wrist pain. J Hand Surg [Br] 1997;22:714–8.

[107] Zanetti M, Bram J, Hodler J. Triangular fibrocartilage and intercarpal ligaments of the wrist: does MR arthrography improve standard MRI? J Magn Reson Imaging 1997;7:590–4.

[108] Potter HG, Asnis-Ernberg L, Weiland AJ, et al. The utility of high-resolution magnetic resonance imaging in the evaluation of the triangular fibrocartilage complex of the wrist. J Bone Joint Surg Am 1997;79:1675–84.

[109] Kato H, Nakamura R, Shionoya K, et al. Does high-resolution MR imaging have better accuracy than standard MR imaging for evaluation of the triangular fibrocartilage complex? J Hand Surg [Br] 2000;25B:487–91.

[110] Saupe N, Prussmann KP, Luechinger R, et al. MR imaging of the wrist: comparison between 1.5- and 3T MR imaging—preliminary experience. Radiology 2005;234:256–64.

[111] Yoshioka H, Ueno T, Tanaka T, et al. High-resolution MR imaging of triangular fibrocartilage complex (TFCC): comparison of microscopy coils and a conventional small surface coil. Skeletal Radiol 2003;32:575–81.

[112] Lenk S, Ludescher B, Martirosan P, et al. 3T high-resolution MR imaging of the carpal ligaments and TFCC. Rofo 2004;176:664–7.

[113] Braun H, Kenn W, Schneider S, et al. Direct MR arthrography of the wrist- value in detecting complete and partial defects of intrinsic ligaments and the TFCC in comparison with arthroscopy. Rofo 2003;175:1515–24.

[114] Meier R, Schmitt R, Krimmer H. Wrist lesions in MRI arthrography compared with wrist arthroscopy. Handchir Mikrochir Plast Chir 2005; 37:85–9.

[115] Schmitt R, Christopoulos G, Meier R, et al. Direct MR arthrography of the wrist in comparison with arthroscopy: a prospective study on 125 patients. Rofo 2003;175:911–9.

[116] Schweitzer ME, Brahme SK, Hodler J, et al. Chronic wrist pain: spin-echo and short tau inversion recovery MR imaging and conventional and MR arthrography. Radiology 1992;182:205–11.

[117] Herold T, Lenhart M, Held P, et al. Indirect MR arthrography of the wrist in the diagnosis of TFCC-lesions. Rofo 2001;173:1006–11.

[118] Scheck RJ, Kubitzek C, Hierner R, et al. The scapholunate interosseous ligament in MR arthrography of the wrist: correlation with non-enhanced MRI and wrist arthroscopy. Skeletal Radiol 1997;26:263–71.

[119] Schadel-Hopfner M, Iwinska-Zelder J, Braus T, et al. MRI versus arthroscopy in the diagnosis of scapholunate ligament injury. J Hand Surg [Br] 2001;26:17–21.

[120] Meier R, Schmitt R, Christopoulos G, et al. Scapholunate ligament tears in MR arthrography compared with wrist arthroscopy. Handchir Mikrochir Plast Chir 2002;34:381–5.

[121] Watson RM, Roach NA, Dalinka MK. Avascular necrosis and bone marrow edema syndrome. Radiol Clin North Am 2004;42:207–19.

[122] Newberg AH, Newman JS. Imaging the painful hip. Clin Orthop Relat Res 2003;406:19–28.

[123] Schmid MR, Notzli HP, Zanetti M, et al. Cartilage lesions in the hip: diagnostic effectiveness of MR arthrography. Radiology 2003;226: 382–6.

[124] Edwards DJ, Lomas D, Villar RN. Diagnosis of the painful hip by magnetic resonance imaging and arthroscopy. J Bone Joint Surg Br 1995; 77:374–6.

[125] Hodler J, Trudell D, Pathria MN, et al. Width of the articular cartilage of the hip: quantification by using fat-suppression spin-echo MR imaging in cadavers. AJR Am J Roentgenol 1992; 159:351–5.

[126] Nishii T, Sugano N, Sato Y, et al. Three-dimensional distribution of acetabular cartilage thickness in patients with hip dysplasia: a fully automated computational analysis of MR imaging. Osteoarthritis Cartilage 2004;12:650–7.

[127] Nakanishi K, Tanaka H, Sugano N, et al. MR-based three-dimensional presentation of cartilage thickness in the femoral head. Eur Radiol 2001;11:2178–83.

[128] Mintz DN, Hooper T, Connell D, et al. Magnetic resonance imaging of the hip: detection of labral and chondral abnormalities using noncontrast imaging. Arthroscopy 2005;21: 385–93.

[129] Bencardino JT, Kassarjian A, Palmer WE. Magnetic resonance imaging of the hip: sports-related injuries. Top Magn Reson Imaging 2003; 14:145–60.

[130] Keeney JA, Peelle MW, Jackson J, et al. Magnetic resonance arthrography versus arthroscopy in the evaluation of articular hip pathology. Clin Orthop Relat Res 2004;429:163–9.

[131] Knuesel PR, Pfirrmann CW, Noetzli HP, et al. MR arthrography of the hip: diagnostic performance of a dedicated water-excitation 3D double-echo steady-state sequence to detect cartilage lesions. AJR Am J Roentgenol 2004; 183:1729–35.

[132] Rubin SJ, Totterman SM, Meyers SP, et al. Magnetic resonance imaging of the hip with a pelvic phased-array surface coil: a technical note. Skeletal Radiol 1998;27:77–82.

[133] Ito K, Leunig M, Ganz R. Histopathologic features of the acetabular labrum in femoroacetabular impingement. Clin Orthop Relat Res 2004; 429:262–71.

[134] Leunig M, Podeszwa D, Beck M, et al. Magnetic resonance arthrography of labral disorders in hips with dysplasia and impingement. Clin Orthop Relat Res 2004;418:74–80.

[135] Narvani AA, Tsiridis E, Kendall S, et al. A preliminary report on prevalence of acetabular labrum tears in sports patients with groin pain. Knee Surg Sports Traumatol Arthrosc 2003; 11:403–8.

[136] Kelley B, Anderson R, Miles K. Acetabular labrum tear in a 15-year-old male: diagnosis with correlative imaging. Australas Radiol 1997; 41:157–9.

[137] Czerny C, Oschatz E, Neuhold A, et al. MR arthrography of the hip joint. Radiologe 2002; 42:451–6.

[138] Czerny C, Kramer J, Neuhold A, et al. Magnetic resonance imaging and magnetic resonance arthrography of the acetabular labrum: comparison with surgical findings. Rofo 2001;173:702–7.

[139] Palmer WE. MR arthrography of the hip. Semin Musculoskelet Radiol 1998;2:349–62.

[140] Kijowski R, Tuite M, Sanford M. Magnetic resonance imaging of the elbow. Part II: abnormalities of the ligaments, tendons, and nerves. Skeletal Radiol 2005;34:1–18.

[141] Melloni P, Valls R. The use of MRI scanning for investigating soft-tissue abnormalities in the elbow. Eur J Radiol 2005;54:303–13.

[142] Kaplan LJ, Potter HG. MR imaging of ligament injuries to the elbow. Magn Reson Imaging Clin N Am 2004;12:221–32.

[143] Timmerman LA, Schwartz ML, Andrews JR. Preoperative evaluation of the ulnar collateral ligament by magnetic resonance imaging and computed tomography arthrography. Evaluation in 25 baseball players with surgical confirmation. Am J Sports Med 1994;22: 26–31.

[144] Cotten A, Jacobsen J, Brossman J, et al. Collateral ligaments of the elbow: conventional MR imaging and MR arthrography with coronal oblique plane and elbow flexion. Radiology 1997; 204:806–12.

[145] Cotten A, Jacobson J, Brossmann J, et al. MR arthrography of the elbow: normal anatomy and diagnostic pitfalls. J Comput Assist Tomogr 1997;21:516–22.

[146] Nakanishi K, Masatomi T, Ochi T, et al. MR arthrography of elbow: evaluation of the ulnar collateral ligament of elbow. Skeletal Radiol 1996;25:629–34.

[147] Carrino JA, Morrison WB, Zou KH, et al. Lateral ulnar collateral ligament of the elbow: optimization of evaluation with two-dimensional MR imaging. Radiology 2001;218:118–25.

[148] Carrino JA, Morrison WB, Zou KH, et al. Noncontrast MR imaging and MR arthrography of the ulnar collateral ligament of the elbow: prospective evaluation of two-dimensional pulse sequences for detection of complete tears. Skeletal Radiol 2001;30:625–32.

[149] Yoshioka H, Ueno T, Tanaka T, et al. High-resolution MR imaging of the elbow using a microscopy surface coil and a clinical 1.5T MR machine: preliminary results. Skeletal Radiol 2004;33:265–71.

[150] Klein MA. MR imaging of the ankle: normal and abnormal findings in the medial collateral ligament. AJR Am J Roentgenol 1994;162:377–83.

[151] Cova M, Assante M, Frezza F, et al. [Magnetic resonance of tibiotalar and subtalar joints Normal anatomy.] Radiol Med (Torino) 1995; 89:203–10. [in Italian].

[152] Rosenberg ZS, Bencardino J, Astion D, et al. MRI features of chronic injuries of the superior peroneal retinaculum. AJR Am J Roentgenol 2003;181:1551–7.

[153] Schaffler GJ, Tirman PF, Stoller DW, et al. Impingement syndrome of the ankle following supination external rotation trauma: MR imaging findings with arthroscopic correlation. Eur Radiol 2003;13:1357–62.

[154] Lektrakul N, Chung CB, Lai YM, et al. Tarsal sinus: arthrographic, MR imaging, MR arthrographic, and pathologic findings in cadavers and retrospective study data in patients with sinus tarsi syndrome. Radiology 2001;219:802–10.

[155] Fiorella D, Helms CA, Nunley JA II. The MR imaging features of the posterior intermalleolar ligament in patients with posterior impingement syndrome of the ankle. Skeletal Radiol 1999;28:573–6.

[156] Farooki S, Yao L, Seeger LL. Anterolateral impingement of the ankle: effectiveness of MR imaging. Radiology 1998;207:357–60.

[157] Breitenseher MJ, Trattnig S, Kukla C, et al. MRI versus lateral stress radiography in acute lateral ankle ligament injuries. J Comput Assist Tomogr 1997;21:280–5.

[158] Verhaven EF, Shahabpour M, Handelberg FW, et al. The accuracy of three-dimensional magnetic resonance imaging in the diagnosis of ruptures of the lateral ligaments of the ankle. Am J Sports Med 1991;19: 583–7.

[159] Breitenseher MJ, Trattnig S, Kukla C, et al. Injuries to the lateral ligaments of the ankle joint: study technic and demonstration by means of MRI. Rofo 1996;164:226–32.

[160] Muhle C, Frank LR, Rand T, et al. Collateral ligaments of the ankle: high-resolution MR imaging with a local gradient coil and anatomic correlation in cadavers. Radiographics 1999; 19:673–83.

[161] Oae K, Takao M, Naito K, et al. Injury to the tibiofibular syndesmosis: value of MR imaging for diagnosis. Radiology 2003;227:155–61.

[162] Takao M, Ochi M, Oae K, et al. Diagnosis of a tear of the tibiofibular syndesmosis. The role of arthroscopy of the ankle. J Bone Joint Surg Br 2003;85:324–9.

[163] Muhle C, Frank LR, Rand T, et al. Tibiofibular syndesmosis: high-resolution MRI using a local gradient coil. J Comput Assist Tomogr 1998;22: 938–44.

MAGNETIC
RESONANCE
IMAGING CLINICS

Magn Reson Imaging Clin N Am (2006) 63–76

Musculoskeletal Imaging at 3T: Current Techniques and Future Applications

Timothy J. Mosher MD

- Technical considerations
- Standard clinical imaging
  Knee imaging
  Hip imaging at 3T
  Shoulder imaging
- *Small joint imaging*
- Emerging techniques of 3T
  musculoskeletal MR imaging
- Summary
- References

Since 2003, human clinical 3T MR imaging platforms have been one of the fastest growing sectors of the MR imaging market. Although the push to higher magnetic field strength was driven initially by neuroimaging applications—in particular functional MR imaging, where there is a specific need to maximize susceptibility-based contrast—application of this technology has extended quickly into all fields of clinical MR imaging. In part, because of the rapid development of ultrahigh-field clinical MR imaging, few controlled studies have evaluated diagnostic efficacy of this new technology. For the most part, clinical experience with 3T MR imaging is anecdotal and unpublished. Despite a lack of evidence to indicate superiority or even equivalency with existing 1.5T scanners and the added cost that can exceed $1 million, clinical 3T MR imaging instrumentation can be found in a variety of settings, from the research laboratory to the community outpatient practice.

The higher signal-to-noise ratio (SNR) that is available with 3T provides the potential to increase diagnostic accuracy through improved image quality. This may come in the form of higher spatial resolution, speed, or optimization of contrast that

is SNR limited (eg, diffusion weighting), or contrast mechanisms (eg, $T2^*$) that are dependent on field strength. In the case of musculoskeletal (MSK) applications, higher SNR is used primarily to increase imaging speed or spatial resolution; however, for many indications it is not clear that improved image quality leads to improved diagnostic accuracy. For example, previous studies that evaluated the effect of field strength on diagnostic accuracy found no difference between low-field scanners (<0.5T) and 1.5T instruments in the diagnosis of anterior cruciate ligament (ACL) tears and meniscal tears [1–3], although high-field strength images may improve diagnostic confidence [4]. Similarly, field strength has not been demonstrated to influence accuracy in the diagnosis of rotator cuff [5–8], or labral and capsular pathology in the shoulder [9]. In the evaluation of small joints of the hands, low-field dedicated extremity scanners have demonstrated diagnostic efficacy that is similar to that of high-field (1T) platforms for the detection of synovitis and joint erosion [10,11]. A common limitation of these studies is that they generally were uncontrolled and retrospective, and frequently compared optimized low-field dedicated extremity

Department of Radiology, Penn State Milton S. Hershey Medical Center, MC H066, 500 University Drive, Hershey, PA 17033, USA
E-mail address: tmosher@psu.edu

scanners. Based on this experience, it is unlikely that diagnostic accuracy for these conditions will be improved substantially with the transition from 1.5T to 3T. For these common indications, diagnostic accuracy is high and does not seem to be limited by factors that are related to SNR efficiency. For these studies, the relative advantage of 3T needs to come in the form of faster imaging time while maintaining an equivalent level of contrast resolution; however, there are indications in which accurate diagnosis seems limited by the available SNR. Some investigators demonstrated lower diagnostic accuracy in the evaluation of the shoulder, particularly labral pathology [12,13]; evaluation of early cartilage lesions [1,14–16]; preoperative spine assessment [17]; or small ligaments [18,19] where diagnostic accuracy is lower at lower field strength. In other situations, such as bilateral hip evaluations or peripheral nerve lesions, current MR imaging studies at 1.5T are challenging because of the simultaneous need for large field-of-view (FOV) coverage and high spatial resolution, which is needed to resolve small structures (eg, acetabular labrum). For these applications, a higher SNR allows acquisition of high-image matrices while effectively using techniques, such as parallel imaging or partial Fourier acquisition, to maintain reasonable image acquisition times. Finally the higher SNR that is available at 3T may lead to new MSK applications of MR imaging that are not feasible at lower field strength, such as new forms of image contrast [20,21], nonproton MR imaging [22], and functional MSK MR imaging applications [23].

In this article, techniques for optimizing 3T MSK MR imaging are reviewed, along with methods for minimizing image artifact. Current clinical experience with standard MR imaging protocols is reviewed, and illustrated with case examples. Finally, emerging applications of ultrahigh-field MSK MR imaging is presented.

Technical considerations

For frequencies less than 250 MHz, SNR increases linearly with field strength [24,25]. Thus, with all other parameters being equal, 3T has the potential to double SNR relative to 1.5T. The field strength dependency of SNR is counterbalanced by the frequency dependency of relaxation times, and the need to alter image acquisition parameters (eg, receiver bandwidth, pulse parameters) to reduce image artifact, and to maintain radiofrequency heating within US Food and Drug Administration (FDA)-regulated limits for specific absorption rate (SAR). As a result, the actual improvement in SNR is less than the theoretic factor of two, and is tissue- and pulse sequence–dependent. For example, in a study on cadaver knees that compared the SNR of T1 (spin lattice relaxation time)-weighted spin-echo images at 3T with that obtained at 1T, the increase in SNR ranged from 39% to 79% [26], significantly less than the three-fold increase that was predicted. In a comparison of T1-weighted fat-suppressed spoiled gradient echo (SPGR) images that were optimized for visualization of articular cartilage, the improvement in SNR at 3T compared with 1.5T ranged from 40% for fluid to 65% for articular cartilage [27].

The potential increase in SNR at 3T is offset, in part, by the frequency dependency of T1. As summarized in Table 1, the T1 of MSK tissues increases by 10% to 30% by moving from 1.5T to 3T. For

Table 1:	Field dependence of T1 and T2 for musculoskeletal tissue				
	T1 (seconds)		**T2 (seconds)**		
Tissue	*1.5T*	*3T*	*1.5T*	*3T*	Reference
Muscle	0.98	1.83 (4 T)	0.031	0.026 (4 T)	Duewell et al [28]
	1.13	1.42	0.035	0.032	Gold et al [48]
	0.86	0.90	0.027	0.029	de Bazelaire et al [62]
	1.03	1.41	0.044	0.050	Stanisz et al [31]
Fat	0.31	0.39 (4 T)	0.047	0.038 (4 T)	Duewell et al [28]
	0.29	0.37	0.17	0.13	Gold et al [48]
	0.34	0.38	0.058	0.068	de Bazelaire et al [62]
Bone marrow	0.29	0.42 (4 T)	0.047	0.044 (4 T)	Duewell et al [28]
	0.29	0.37	0.17	0.13	Gold et al [48]
	0.55	0.59	0.049	0.049	de Bazelaire et al [62]
Cartilage	0.77	1.39 (4 T)	0.039	0.025 (4 T)	Duewell et al [28]
	1.06	1.24	0.042	0.037	Gold et al [48]
	1.02	1.17	0.030	0.027	Stanisz et al [31]
Synovial fluid	1.47	5.71 (4 T)	0.535	0.207 (4 T)	Duewell et al [28]
	2.85	3.62	1.21	0.77	Gold et al [48]

a constant time to repetition (TR) value, the increase in saturation that results from the longer T1 values can negate the increase in SNR at the higher field strength [28]. To maintain T1-weighted contrast that is equivalent to 1.5T, it is necessary to increase TR. This is less of a problem for imaging of joints that rely heavily on proton density (PD)–weighted images with the longer TR value determined by the number of slices that is needed to provide adequate coverage. In cases of bone marrow or soft tissue imaging in which T1-weighted imaging is needed, the author typically increases TR values by 20% relative to that used at 1.5T.

In contrast to T1, T2 (spin-spin relaxation time) values remain constant or decrease slightly with increasing field strength [29]. The observed field dependency of T2 is influenced by tissue type, pulse sequence, and acquisition parameters. With increasing B0 (static magnetic field strength), there is a linear increase in microscopic magnetic field gradients that is produced by tissue domains with different magnetic susceptibility. For MSK imaging, these gradients are largest in tissues, such as bone marrow, or the tidemark region of articular cartilage that contains a mixture of calcified and noncalcified tissue. Significant susceptibility-induced gradients also are present in tissue that contains paramagnetic metals, such as blood degradation products. Diffusion of water molecules through these gradients leads to T2 relaxation. The influence of diffusion on the observed T2 increases with longer echo-spacing and size of the susceptibility-induced gradients. Increasing time to echo (TE) or interecho spacing in fast spin echo (FSE) sequences increases the time for diffusion to occur, and thereby, decreases T2. The diffusion term scales with the second power of the gradient strength; thus the effect of diffusion through these magnetic field gradients at 3T is four times greater than at 1.5T. As a result, with increasing field strength there is coupling of T2* and T2 contrast [30].

The effect of field strength on image contrast is more apparent in T2* contrast that is generated by gradient-echo techniques. The absence of a 180° refocusing pulse does not allow for refocusing of the phase dispersion that is produced by static magnetic field gradients; this leads to substantial shortening of T2* at 3T. This can result in image artifact (eg, loss of signal from the deep layer of articular cartilage), which may lead to an underestimation of cartilage thickness. The short T2* contrast also is apparent in bone marrow, which generally is hypointense on gradient-echo images that are obtained at 3T. The increased sensitivity to susceptibility should be considered in diagnostic interpretation of spine MR imaging, because calcification of ligaments, osteophytes, or uncovertebral joint hypertrophy may

lead to overestimation of the degree of stenosis. This sensitivity to susceptibility-induced magnetic field gradients is illustrated in Fig. 1. As opposed to T1 and T2 contrast, which have field strength dependence, magnetization transfer, another important mechanism of contrast for MSK MR imaging, is independent of field strength [31].

Fat suppression is a central component of MSK MR imaging, and is necessary for accurate characterization of bone marrow pathology, soft tissue inflammation, and identification of contrast enhancement. Because chemical shift scales linearly with field strength, the separation of the fat and water resonances at 3T is twice that at 1.5T. This allows for more complete suppression of the fat peak without spurious saturation of the water peak. Because of greater fat–water separation, the length of the fat suppression pulse can be shortened, which allows shorter TR values or additional slices to be acquired for a set TR. In addition, the longer T1 of fat at 3T allows less recovery of longitudinal magnetization between the chemical shift selective fat suppression pulse and image acquisition, and thereby, provides more complete fat suppression. In the author's experience, fat suppression at 3T can be too complete and leads to loss of anatomic margins between fat and hypointense tissue (eg, tendons, ligaments). For these cases, the degree of fat suppression can be tailored using partial fat suppression techniques.

The field dependence of chemical shift also must be considered in terms of chemical shift artifact. This is particularly important in MSK MR imaging where it is necessary to visualize clearly the margins of tissues (eg, cartilage, tendon) that are adjacent to fatty tissues. As illustrated in Fig. 2, using acquisition parameters that are appropriate for 1.5T results in chemical shift artifact that completely obscures cartilage. The degree of misregistration that is produced by the difference in chemical shift is a function of field strength and receiver bandwidth. The chemical shift scales linearly with B0. To maintain the same level of chemical shift artifact at 3T that is present at 1.5T, it is necessary to double the receiver bandwidth. Because SNR is inversely proportional to the square root of the receiver bandwidth, this lowers SNR by the square root of two, or 44%. For cases, such as joint imaging, in which chemical shift artifact must be minimized to visualize important structures, the need for high receiver bandwidth partially offsets the greater SNR provided at 3T. For cases in which it is possible to use fat suppression techniques, or situations where chemical shift artifact does not impact diagnosis, smaller bandwidths may be used, which thereby recover a greater portion of the increased SNR that is possible at 3T.

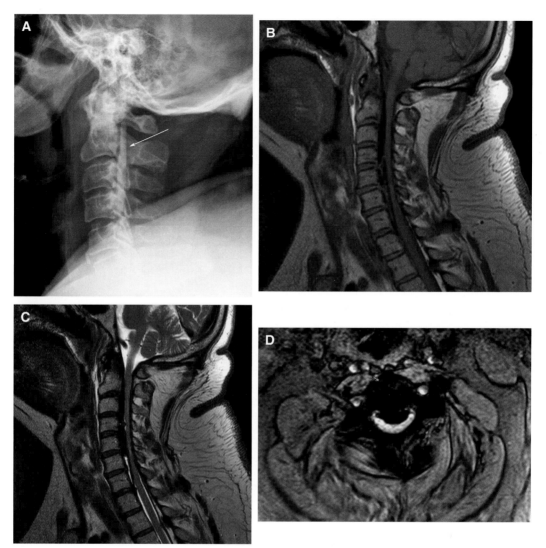

Figure 1 (*A*) 59-year-old man presented with progressive symptoms of cervical myelopathy secondary to ossification of the posterior longitudinal ligament (*arrow*) demonstrated on lateral cervical spine radiograph. (*B*) Sagittal 3T T1-weighted FSE (TR/TE: 600 milliseconds/7 milliseconds) and (*C*) T2-weighted FSE (TR/TE: 5000 milliseconds/110 milliseconds) images confirm marked cervical canal stenosis. (*D*) Sensitivity of 3T T2*-weighted gradient echo (TR/TE: 480 milliseconds/12 milliseconds) image to macroscopic gradients produced by differences in tissue magnetic susceptibility produces blooming artifact that accentuates the degree of stenosis.

Along with chemical shift artifact, artifact from metallic orthopedic hardware is encountered frequently in MSK MR imaging, and is more severe at 3T. Differences in bulk magnetic susceptibility of metal and tissue generate static magnetic field gradients that increase linearly with B0. The orientation and magnitude of susceptibility-induced field gradients is influenced further by the geometry and orientation of the device with respect to the applied magnetic field. Depending on the size of the susceptibility-induced gradient, the artifact may appear as geometric distortion of the image or a signal void. Geometric distortion is apparent on spin-echo

and gradient-echo techniques as bands of increased and decreased signal intensity. This artifact occurs when gradients that are generated by susceptibility differences between paramagnetic metal, such as stainless steel, and diamagnetic tissue distort the linearity of the slice or frequency-encoding gradient. As a result of the nonlinearity, the voxel geometry is no longer equal across the image.

Geometric distortion also occurs near the periphery of the magnet bore or with large FOV images as a result of nonlinearity of the spatially encoding gradients. This artifact is more pronounced on short-bore 3T systems and can limit the FOV in

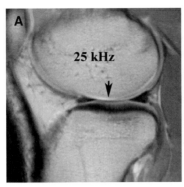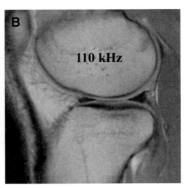

Figure 2 Chemical shift artifact at 3T. (*A*) Sagittal T1-weighted SE image obtained with a receiver bandwidth of 25 kHz results in a fat/water separation of seven pixels. Chemical shift artifact from subchondral bone marrow is superimposed on the femoral articular cartilage (*arrow*). (*B*) Increasing the receiver bandwidth to 110 kHz decreases the chemical shift to 1.5 pixels.

some applications, particularly when the region of interest is away from the center of the magnetic field gradients. This is a diagnostic limitation in MSK oncologic imaging that often requires large longitudinal FOVs to cover joint to joint. On some systems, this artifact is corrected, in part, by using postprocessing algorithms that adjust for gradient nonlinearity.

The signal void that is produced by susceptibility artifact is caused by phase dispersion that results from local magnetic field gradients that are produced by differences in magnetic susceptibility between the two materials. The magnitude of these gradients increases linearly with magnetic field strength, and is most severe with gradient-echo techniques. Although FSE or short TE spin-echo techniques reduce the artifact, diffusion of protons through the gradient leads to signal loss on gradient and spin-echo images. Thus, to minimize signal void, the interecho spacing must be minimized, which necessitates high bandwidth and rapid gradient switching. This should be done with caution.

Depending on the orientation of the hardware, rapid gradient switching may induce eddy currents in the metal that may worsen the artifact and increase the degree of geometric distortion.

A recent review highlighted practical approaches to MR imaging in the setting of metal hardware [32]. Careful screening of patients before imaging on the 3T scanner is a critical first step in acquiring diagnostic images. The author avoids scanning patients with stainless steel hardware in the vicinity of the region of interest on the 3T scanner. As illustrated in Fig. 3, with proper technique, artifact from hardware can be minimized and can result in high-quality diagnostic images at 3T. First, gradient-echo imaging techniques lead to substantially larger artifact and should be avoided. Fast spin-echo proton density– or T1-weighted images are preferred because they reduce signal loss from diffusion, and refocus the phase dispersion that is caused by the static field gradients that are generated near metal implants. Second, the use a high receiver bandwidth setting and a large image matrix, and

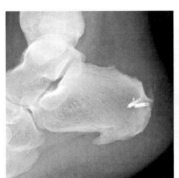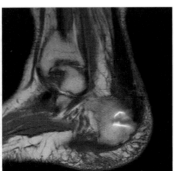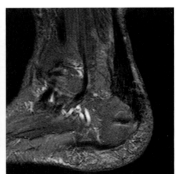

Figure 3 Susceptibility artifact. Patient with a history of resection of a Haglund's deformity and reimplantation of the Achilles tendon with stainless steel tendon anchors. Sagittal T1 and T2 fat-suppressed FSE MR imaging at 3T using high receiver bandwidth demonstrate minimal susceptibility artifact that allows diagnostic visualization of the tendon insertion.

reduction of the interecho spacing further reduce the artifact. Third, when possible, the long axis of the hardware should be positioned parallel to the direction of the main magnetic field and the direction of the frequency-encoding axis should be directed away from the region of interest. Around curved components it is useful to acquire two separate images, swapping the frequency and phase-encoding directions to allow circumferential visualization of tissue around spherical components, such as joint prosthesis. Fourth, in certain cases, it is useful to obtain fluid-sensitive sequences to evaluate for bone marrow edema, joint effusion, or periarticular fluid collections. In this setting, the short tau inversion recovery technique is preferred because it is less sensitive to magnetic field inhomogeneity than are chemical shift selective fat suppression techniques.

In addition to screening patients for the presence of implanted devices to identify potential sources of image artifact, it is critical to identify potential devices or conditions that may pose a safety hazard. Most medical devices that are deemed MR imaging safe or compatible were designed and tested for field strengths up to 1.5T. Devices that are safe at 1.5T should not be assumed to be safe at 3T; they require additional ex vivo testing. Testing of these devices is ongoing. The policy at the author's institution is to exclude individuals with devices that are not verified to be MR imaging safe at 3T or higher. In addition to deflection or torque of implants from the static field, there is risk from radiofrequency (RF) heating. In theory, the RF power that is deposited within the body increases quadratically with B0. In actuality, it seems that the power deposited is less than the fourfold increase that is predicted when going from 1.5T to 3T [30]. This is for bulk soft tissue power deposition. Local power deposition [33], particularly around conductive implants, may be higher. For patients with conductive implants, it is recommended to perform MR imaging studies under reduced power settings.

For RF-intensive pulse sequences, such as FSE, acquisition parameters often need to be adjusted to maintain the SAR at less than the FDA limit. This may entail reducing the number of slices, or increasing TR. A simple approach is to reduce the refocusing pulse to less than 180° [34], which reduces RF power deposition with a moderate reduction in signal intensity. Techniques, such as transition between pseudosteady states (TRAPS) [35,36] or hyperechoes [37], are particularly effective for modulating the power of the 180°-refocusing pulse to maximize SNR efficiency while reducing RF power deposition. With these techniques it is possible to reduce RF power by a factor of 2.5 to 6 without a loss in signal intensity [36],

and to maintain the high signal acquisition efficiency, with echo train lengths at 3T that are comparable to those used at 1.5T. Alternatively, RF power may be reduced by using hybrid techniques, such as GRASE [38], that combine spin-echoes and gradient echoes to fill k-space. Depending on how the gradient and spin-echoes are acquired, this approach can alter image contrast through additional $T2^*$ contrast, and may cause signal dropout at fat/water interfaces, if gradient echoes are acquired out of phase.

Standard clinical imaging

Knee imaging

With the high availability of clinical 3T phased array extremity coils, early clinical experience at 3T has been greatest with knee MR imaging. Given the high reliance of MSK MR imaging on proton density–weighted imaging for most joint protocols, the transition from 1.5T to 3T has been straight-forward for MSK radiologists. For collagen-rich tissues (eg, tendons, ligaments, menisci), image contrast is dominated by the short T2 ($\sim$250 µs) [39], which is essentially independent of field strength, and is affected minimally by TR. Diagnostic findings, such as whether a tendon is normal, degenerated, or torn, are differentiated by short TE or long TE sequences, and are similar between the two field strengths. This is not true for MR imaging examinations in other areas of the body, such as the brain, where there is greater reliance on T1-weighted contrast. The tendency for T1 values of tissues to converge at higher field strength leads to a loss of T1 contrast with standard techniques at 3T. This can be a source of consternation for neuroradiologists as they make the transition to 3T.

At the author's institution, the knee MR imaging protocols are nearly identical at 1.5T and 3T, with the exception of reducing the number of averages at the higher field strength. In addition, the receiver bandwidth is doubled to maintain equivalent chemical shift artifact and the TRAPS technique is implemented to reduce RF power. For axial fat-suppressed imaging, the TE at 3T is reduced from 38 milliseconds to 30 milliseconds, and images are acquired with a 512 matrix to enhance contrast resolution from articular cartilage. With these simple modifications, the author routinely obtains high-quality diagnostic images at slightly lower total imaging times. Examples are illustrated in Figs. 4 through 7.

Hip imaging at 3T

Clinical MR imaging evaluation of the hip presents unique challenges to the MSK radiologist. Many patients have nonspecific symptoms that are difficult

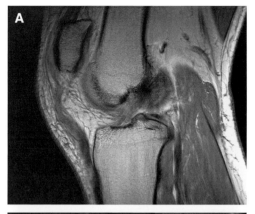

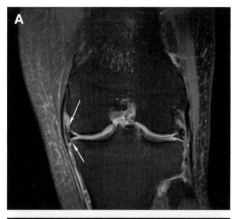

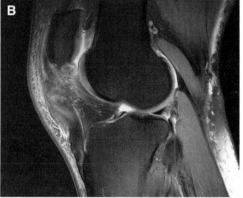

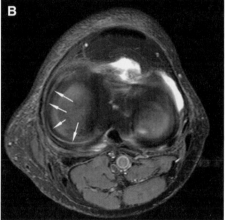

Figure 4 32-year-old man with extensor weakness after a fall. (*A*) Sagittal FSE PD-weighted (TR/TE: 2875 milliseconds/15 milliseconds) and (*B*) FSE PD-weighted (TR/TE: 3000 milliseconds/30 milliseconds) fat-suppressed 3T MR imaging demonstrates avulsion of the patellar tendon from the inferior patellar pole with patella alta. A complete patellar tendon tear was repaired at surgery.

Figure 5 3T knee MR imaging in a 53-year-old with knee pain after a fall. (*A*) Coronal (TR/TE: 2150 milliseconds/30 milliseconds) and (*B*) axial (TR/TE: 1500 milliseconds/30 milliseconds) FSE PD images with fat suppression demonstrate a large peripheral tear of the medial meniscus (*arrows*) that extends from the posterior to the anterior horn of the medial meniscus. The examination also demonstrated a complete ACL disruption and horizontal cleavage tear of the lateral meniscus.

to localize. Symptoms may be a result of systemic processes that may affect both hips (eg, avascular necrosis) to focal internal hip derangement (eg, labral pathology). This necessitates anatomic coverage over a large region, frequently the entire pelvis. Thus, there is the conflicting requirement for large FOV while maintaining high spatial resolution to visualize critical soft tissue structures adequately. This requires large image matrices, which leads to long image acquisition times with conventional acquisition methods. Hip MR imaging evaluation is even more challenging because of the deep location in the body, which limits selection of appropriate surface coils and reduces available SNR. Because of lower SNR at 1.5T and the need for signal averaging to maintain sufficient image quality for diagnosis, techniques, such as parallel imaging or half Fourier imaging, are ineffective means of reducing imaging times. A major advantage of the higher SNR that is available at 3T is the potential to use parallel imaging or partial Fourier acquisition techniques efficiently to obtain images that have a large FOV and high spatial resolution in a reasonable scan time.

Of particular interest is the use of 3T MR imaging in the evaluation of the acetabular labrum and hip cartilage. There is growing recognition of conditions, such as femoral acetabular impingement, which can be a source of hip pain in younger adults and is a risk factor for premature hip osteoarthritis. With development of new surgical treatment options, such as disarticulation femoral head/neck osteoplasty, there is a need for accurate preoperative diagnosis. In addition to abnormal femoral head neck morphology, the condition is characterized by anterior superior acetabular labral tears and

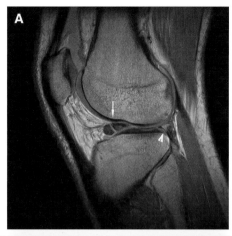

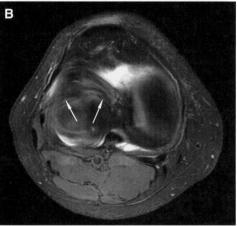

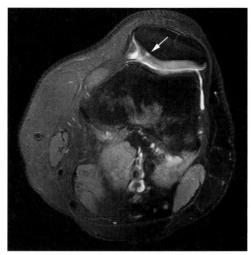

Figure 7 19-year-old man with retropatellar knee pain that was unresponsive to conservative therapy. The FSE PD-weighted (TR/TE: 3850 milliseconds/30 milliseconds) fat suppressed axial 3T MR imaging demonstrates a full thickness fissure of the medial patellar facet with high signal at the bone/cartilage interface, which is suggestive of a delamination injury (*arrow*). Arthroscopy confirmed a linear chondral fracture with a 1-cm segment of delaminated articular cartilage that was treated with chondroplasty.

Figure 6 24-year-old with lateral knee pain and locking after a recent injury. (*A*) Sagittal PD-weighted image (TR/TE: 2880 milliseconds/15 milliseconds) demonstrates a flipped posterior horn of the lateral meniscus (*arrow*). The residual inferior meniscopopliteal fascicle is still identified (*arrowhead*). (*B*) The axial FSE PD image (TR/TE: 4050 milliseconds/30 milliseconds) confirms the large bucket handle tear with anterior location of the flipped posterior horn (*arrows*).

articular cartilage defects [40–42]. MR arthrography provides high accuracy for the diagnosis of labral tears (90–95%) [41,43,44], whereas sensitivity for the detection of cartilage lesions in the hip is variable (50–95%) [44–46]. In general, the diagnostic accuracy for hip cartilage is substantially lower than that reported in the knee. The curved contour of the thin articular cartilage of the femoral head and a high degree of joint congruity between the acetabular and femoral cartilage makes identification of focal lesions particularly difficult. As illustrated in Figs. 8 and 9, the high-contrast resolution that is available at 3T is particularly useful in the identification of cartilage and labral lesions. Future studies are needed to determine if the perceived

improvement in image quality provides a significant improvement in diagnostic or therapeutic efficacy.

Shoulder imaging

As with the diagnosis of ACL and meniscal tears in the knee, previous studies that evaluated the effect of field strength on diagnostic accuracy found no significant effect in the evaluation of rotator cuff tear. There is potential for improvement in the diagnosis of labral pathology that is limited, in part, by spatial resolution. No published study has evaluated 3T MR imaging in the shoulder, and there is little in the form of pictorial examples of shoulder images [47]. In the author's experience, shoulder MR imaging presents several challenges at 3T. First, for larger patients the shoulder is near the periphery of the magnet bore, which can lead to difficulty in shimming and artifact from geometric distortion for larger FOVs. Second, there can be difficulty with fat suppression because of imperfection in RF homogeneity. This can be corrected partially by using adiabatic pulses for chemical shift fat suppression. Third, 3T is particularly sensitive to motion artifact. This can be a significant problem for patients who have respiratory difficulty.

Small joint imaging

With the development of dedicated surface coils for the imaging of small joints (eg, wrist, finger, elbow,

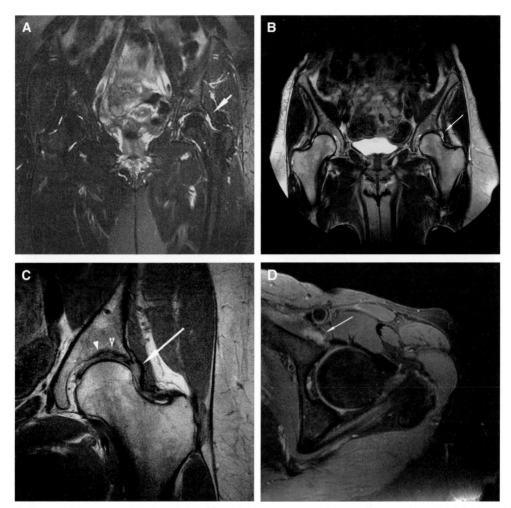

Figure 8 55-year-old woman with chronic left hip pain that was exacerbated with exercise. (*A*) Initial coronal FSE T2-weighted (TR/TE: 4000 milliseconds/110 milliseconds) fat-suppressed image obtained at 1.5T demonstrates fluid signal adjacent to the left superior labrum, which was suggestive of a paralabral cyst (*arrow*). (*B*) Subsequent FSE 3T T2-weighted (TR/TE: 4000 milliseconds/120 milliseconds) image better demonstrates a left paralabral cyst (*arrow*). Geometric distortion from gradient non-linearity is observed at the inferior part of the image (*C*) Localized 3T MR FSE PD-weighted (TR/TE: 200 milliseconds/40 milliseconds) image of the left hip obtained with paired surface coil array demonstrates a cleavage tear of the left superior labrum with an intralabral cyst (*arrow*) and mild degenerative changes of the superior acetabular cartilage (*arrowheads*). (*D*) An anterior paralabral cyst also is identified on the axial FSE PD-weighted (TR/TE: 1300 milliseconds/40 milliseconds) fat-suppressed image (*arrow*).

forefoot), there are likely to be advances in the development of high-resolution imaging at 3T. Current experience suggests that the additional SNR at 3T improves the visualization of critical structures that can be difficult to visualize reproducibly at 1.5T (eg, small intrinsic ligaments of the wrist, small periarticular erosions, articular cartilage). At 1.5T, three-dimensional (3D) gradient-echo techniques are used frequently to provide sufficient spatial resolution to resolve these structures; frequently, this is at the expense of optimal tissue contrast. The lack of significant magnetization transfer

with these techniques can result in increased signal intensity in ligaments and tendons, particularly in older patients who frequently have myxoid degeneration. The increased background signal decreases the ability to visualize discrete tears in these structures. At 3T, it is possible to obtain two-dimensional (2D) FSE images with similar section thickness to that of the 3D sequences that are used at 1.5T. These techniques are reliable methods for visualization of tendon and ligament pathology of large joints, and likely also will improve the diagnosis of pathology in small joints.

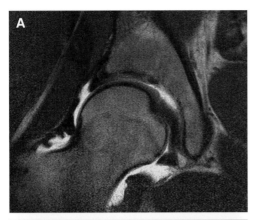

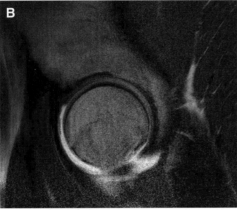

Figure 9 24-year-old woman with pain and popping sensation of right hip with clinical diagnosis of acetabular labral tear. Coronal (*A*) and sagittal (*B*) images from a 3T MR arthrogram of the right hip demonstrate normal contour of the labrum and hip articular cartilage. T1-weighted (TR/TE: 425 milliseconds/15 milliseconds) images were obtained using paired flexible surface coils with a 12-cm FOV and 512^2 acquisition matrix (234-μm pixel resolution). Patient's symptoms improved with conservative therapy.

Emerging techniques of 3T musculoskeletal MR imaging

Evaluation of articular cartilage is the area of MSK imaging that is most likely to benefit from 3T MR imaging. With growing interest in the development and evaluation of new chondroprotective therapies, there is an emerging need to identify early cartilage injury when such treatment is likely to be most effective. Cartilage MR imaging has been a valuable clinical research tool over the past decade; it has become an integral component of large National Institutes of Health–funded multicenter research projects, such as the Osteoarthritis Initiative. As clinicians are becoming more aware of the role of MR imaging in the evaluation of cartilage, there is an increasing demand for radiologists to provide an accurate assessment of cartilage in routine clinical imaging.

The primary MR imaging pulse sequences that are used in evaluating articular cartilage at 1.5T are 3D fat-suppressed T1-weighted spoiled gradient-echo and 2D proton density–weighted fast spin-echo techniques. Each has advantages and disadvantages with respect to contrast resolution and the visualization of articular cartilage.

The major advantage of the 3D T1-weighted gradient-echo techniques is high spatial resolution. This is particularly important in the evaluation of small joints, or curved articular cartilage surfaces (eg, femoral head) where thin sections are needed to delineate cartilage interfaces clearly and minimize volume averaging. Using this technique at 1.5T, it is possible to obtain images with a 1- to 2-mm section thickness and in-plane resolution of 200 to 350 microns per pixel. With 3T, higher SNR may allow these limits to be extended while maintaining sufficient SNR. In addition to improved SNR, it appears that cartilage/fluid contrast is higher at 3T, which thereby, improves the delineation of the articular surface [27,48].

Several disadvantages limit the routine clinical application of 3D gradient-echo techniques at 1.5T. The gradient-echo technique is inefficient for generating contrast resolution, which results in long image acquisition times (6–10 minutes) to acquire a 3D volume of the knee cartilage in the sagittal plane. In 3T applications where there is sufficient SNR, the use of parallel imaging techniques or half-Fourier acquisition can reduce image acquisition times, generally in the range of 33% to 50%, although in theory, greater reduction is possible.

In addition to long acquisition times, standard gradient-echo techniques suffer from poor contrast, which is needed for the evaluation of connective tissues. Although the fat-suppressed T1-weighted gradient-echo technique produces high bulk contrast between cartilage and adjacent tissues that is useful for image segmentation, the lack of substantial magnetization transfer reduces the sensitivity for detection of superficial cartilage lesions and degeneration of the collagen matrix in deeper layers of the tissue. It is poor for the evaluation of other internal derangements (eg, tears of menisci, ligaments, and tendons) and is insensitive to bone marrow pathology.

More recent clinical evaluation of articular cartilage, particularly in the knee, has relied heavily on proton density–weighted FSE images, with or without fat suppression. The primary advantage of this technique is excellent soft tissue contrast with modest image acquisition times of 3 to 4 minutes. The technique also allows for the diagnostic evaluation of critical articular tissues (eg, menisci, bone marrow), which makes it particularly useful in the clinical setting where it is necessary to evaluate the entire joint. The primary disadvantage of the technique is lower spatial resolution; however, this is less of a limitation at 3T where higher SNR can permit higher spatial resolution. Although clinical experience with cartilage at 3T is limited, preliminary results suggest that the higher field strength provides greater diagnostic accuracy in the detection of focal defects [27,49].

New techniques that are based on the steady-state free precession sequence [50,51], and multi-echo T2* sequences [52] have been proposed for cartilage imaging. These techniques provide high-resolution images of cartilage with image contrast that is similar to that obtained with FSE techniques. Although preliminary results are promising, these techniques are not widely available, and have undergone limited validation for routine clinical use.

Initial studies showed improved contrast to noise of the cartilage/bone and cartilage/fluid interface at 3T, compared with 1.5T, for proton density–weighted images (TR/TE = 4000 milliseconds/ 14 milliseconds) [27,48]. This improvement in technical efficacy has led to the greater diagnostic accuracy of 3T in the evaluation of articular cartilage defects. Several initial validation studies compared diagnostic accuracy in the detection of artificial cartilage lesions in excised cartilage specimens.

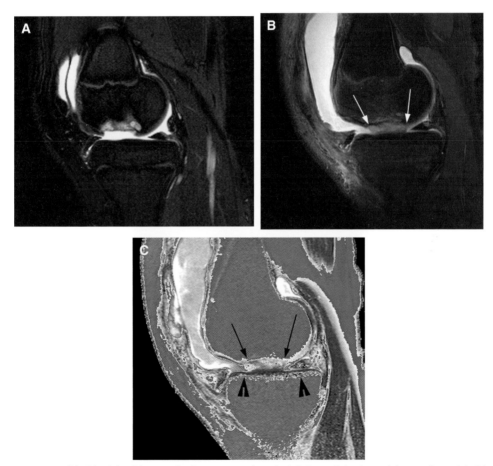

Figure 10 14-year-old girl with a history of a large osteochondral defect of the lateral femoral condyle identified on 1.5T sagittal FSE T2-weighted image (TR/TE: 2950 milliseconds/75 milliseconds) (*A*). The patient subsequently underwent autologous chondrocyte harvesting and implantation (autologous chondrocyte harvesting and implantation [ACI] procedure). (*B*) A 3T fat suppressed FSE T2-weighted (TR/TE: 4550 milliseconds/60 milliseconds) MR imaging obtained 7 months after chondrocyte implantation demonstrates prominent periosteal hypertrophy, and elevated signal in the graft site (*arrows*). (*C*) A cartilage MR imaging T2 map demonstrates heterogeneously elevated cartilage T2 of the graft site consistent with increased water content and loss of normal type II collagen architecture in the cartilage graft (*arrows*). For comparison, normal spatial variation in cartilage T2 is identified in the tibial cartilage with short T2 near the bone, and longer T2 values toward the articular surface (*arrowheads*).

Masi and colleagues [53] found substantially higher accuracy of 3T intermediate-weighted FSE images in comparison to those obtained using an equivalent sequence at 1.5T (90% versus 62%). Similar improvement in the accuracy of diagnosing artificially created osteochondral lesions was obtained using 3T images of talar dome cartilage [54]. A small improvement in the diagnostic accuracy at 3T was observed for fat-suppressed spoiled gradient-echo images (83% versus 79%). In contrast to these results, other investigators found a slight superiority of 3T fat-suppressed 3D-SPGR sequences in the diagnosis of focal cartilage lesions compared with 1.5T [49], but no significant advantage when using fat-saturated proton density–weighted SE sequences [55]. It remains to be determined if the relative improvement in accuracy that is seen with these validation studies is observed in human clinical studies.

A potential area of growth for clinical 3T MR imaging is in the management of patients who have arthritis. In an animal model of inflammatory arthritis, recent laboratory studies demonstrated the potential to use the uptake of small superparamagnetic iron oxide particles in synovial macrophages as a marker of disease activity [56–58]. With the continuing development of effective disease-modifying therapy for inflammatory arthritis, there is a greater need to develop sensitive, noninvasive measures of response to therapy that are prognostic of long-term outcome. Because many of the new therapies are expensive and have potential deleterious side effects, these MR imaging techniques have a potential application in clinical management and in new drug discovery.

The success in development of disease-modifying drugs for inflammatory arthritis has stimulated interest in developing new therapies for modifying osteoarthritis. The application of MR imaging techniques that are sensitive to biochemical and biophysical properties of the extracellular matrix (eg, cartilage T2 mapping (Fig. 10) [59], delayed gadolinium-enhanced MR imaging of cartilage [60]), are being explored as potential image markers of cartilage injury that could be exploited to evaluate the efficacy of new chondroprotective therapy. Recently, these techniques have been applied to the study of cartilage response to exercise [23,61], and have the potential to provide important information on the role of in vivo biomechanics of cartilage, and the effect of exercise on cartilage physiology.

Summary

MSK MR imaging applications are making the transition rapidly from 1.5T to 3T. Initial experience in the knee suggests that the higher SNR provides technical improvement in routine clinical imaging with the potential for greater accuracy in the diagnosis of articular cartilage injury. Similarly, initial experience with 3T MR imaging in the evaluation of the hip and small joints of the hand and wrist has been positive. In other joints, clinical development has been limited by the lack of availability of dedicated surface coils, and sensitivity of 3T MR imaging to artifact. The clinical impact of this technology remains uncertain because no published controlled clinical trial has evaluated the impact of 3T MR imaging on diagnostic outcomes. In addition to clinical application, 3T MR imaging has an important role for furthering translational research in MSK diseases through the development of new molecular and functional MR imaging techniques.

References

[1] Kladny B, Gluckert K, Swoboda B, et al. Comparison of low-field (0.2 Tesla) and high-field (1.5 Tesla) magnetic resonance imaging of the knee joint. Arch Orthop Trauma Surg 1995; 114(5):281–6.

[2] Kersting-Sommerhoff B, Hof N, Lenz M, et al. MRI of peripheral joints with a low-field dedicated system: a reliable and cost-effective alternative to high-field units? Eur Radiol 1996;6(4): 561–5.

[3] Cotten A, Delfaut E, Demondion X, et al. MR imaging of the knee at 0.2 and 1.5 T: correlation with surgery. AJR Am J Roentgenol 2000; 174(4):1093–7.

[4] Rand T, Imhof H, Turetschek K, et al. Comparison of low field (0.2T) and high field (1.5T) MR imaging in the differentiation of torn from intact menisci. Eur J Radiol 1999;30(1):22–7.

[5] Merl T, Scholz M, Gerhardt P, et al. Results of a prospective multicenter study for evaluation of the diagnostic quality of an open whole-body low-field MRI unit. A comparison with high-field MRI measured by the applicable gold standard. Eur J Radiol 1999;30(1):43–53.

[6] Loew R, Kreitner KF, Runkel M, et al. MR arthrography of the shoulder: comparison of low-field (0.2 T) vs high-field (1.5 T) imaging. Eur Radiol 2000;10(6):989–96.

[7] Shellock FG, Bert JM, Fritts HM, et al. Evaluation of the rotator cuff and glenoid labrum using a 0.2-Tesla extremity magnetic resonance (MR) system: MR results compared to surgical findings. J Magn Reson Imaging 2001;14(6):763–70.

[8] Kreitner KF, Loew R, Runkel M, et al. Low-field MR arthrography of the shoulder joint: technique, indications, and clinical results. Eur Radiol 2003;13(2):320–9.

[9] Allmann KH, Walter O, Laubenberger J, et al. Magnetic resonance diagnosis of the anterior labrum and capsule. Effect of field strength on efficacy. Invest Radiol 1998;33(7):415–20.

[10] Taouli B, Zaim S, Peterfy CG, et al. Rheumatoid arthritis of the hand and wrist: comparison of three imaging techniques. AJR Am J Roentgenol 2004;182(4):937–43.

[11] Ejbjerg BJ, Narvestad E, Jacobsen S, et al. Optimised, low cost, low field dedicated extremity MRI is highly specific and sensitive for synovitis and bone erosions in rheumatoid arthritis wrist and finger joints: comparison with conventional high field MRI and radiography. Ann Rheum Dis 2005;64(9):1280–7.

[12] Tung GA, Entzian D, Green A, et al. High-field and low-field MR imaging of superior glenoid labral tears and associated tendon injuries. AJR Am J Roentgenol 2000;174(4):1107–14.

[13] Magee T, Shapiro M, Williams D. Comparison of high-field-strength versus low-field-strength MRI of the shoulder. AJR Am J Roentgenol 2003; 181(5):1211–5.

[14] Verhoek G, Zanetti M, Duewell S, et al. MRI of the foot and ankle: diagnostic performance and patient acceptance of a dedicated low field MR scanner. J Magn Reson Imaging 1998;8(3):711–6.

[15] Ahn JM, Kwak SM, Kang HS, et al. Evaluation of patellar cartilage in cadavers with a low-field-strength extremity-only magnet: comparison of MR imaging sequences, with macroscopic findings as the standard. Radiology 1998; 208(1):57–62.

[16] Harman M, Ipeksoy U, Dogan A, et al. MR arthrography in chondromalacia patellae diagnosis on a low-field open magnet system. Clin Imaging 2003;27(3):194–9.

[17] McCulloch JA. Low-field-strength (open) MRI do not deliver the information needed to plan lumbar microdisectomy and/or microdecompression. Spine J 2001;1(2):160.

[18] Ahn JM, Brown RR, Kwak SM, et al. Evaluation of the triangular fibrocartilage and the scapholunate and lunotriquetral ligaments in cadavers with low-field-strength extremity-only magnet. Comparison of available imaging sequences and macroscopic findings. Invest Radiol 1998;33(7): 401–6.

[19] Rand T, Ahn JM, Muhle C, et al. Ligaments and tendons of the ankle. Evaluation with low-field (0.2 T) MR imaging. Acta Radiol 1999;40(3): 303–8.

[20] Miller KL, Hargreaves BA, Gold GE, et al. Steady-state diffusion-weighted imaging of in vivo knee cartilage. Magn Reson Med 2004;51(2):394–8.

[21] Berg A, Singer T, Moser E. High-resolution diffusivity imaging at 3.0 T for the detection of degenerative changes: a trypsin-based arthritis model. Invest Radiol 2003;38(7):460–6.

[22] Shapiro EM, Borthakur A, Gougoutas A, et al. 23Na MRI accurately measures fixed charge density in articular cartilage. Magn Reson Med 2002; 47(2):284–91.

[23] Mosher TJ, Smith HE, Collins C, et al. Change in knee cartilage T2 at MR imaging after running: a feasibility study. Radiology 2005;234(1):245–9.

[24] Collins CM, Smith MB. Signal-to-noise ratio and absorbed power as functions of main magnetic field strength, and definition of "90 degrees" RF pulse for the head in the birdcage coil. Magn Reson Med 2001;45(4):684–91.

[25] Edelstein WA, Glover GH, Hardy CJ, et al. The intrinsic signal-to-noise ratio in NMR imaging. Magn Reson Med 1986;3(4):604–18.

[26] Niitsu M, Nakai T, Ikeda K, et al. High-resolution MR imaging of the knee at 3.0 T. Acta Radiol 2000;41(1):84–8.

[27] Kornaat PR, Reeder SB, Koo S, et al. MR imaging of articular cartilage at 1.5T and 3.0T: comparison of SPGR and SSFP sequences. Osteoarthritis Cartilage 2005;13(4):338–44.

[28] Duewell SH, Ceckler TL, Ong K, et al. Musculoskeletal MR imaging at 4 T and at 1.5 T: comparison of relaxation times and image contrast. Radiology 1995;196(2):551–5.

[29] Bottomley PA, Foster TH, Argersinger RE, et al. A review of normal tissue hydrogen NMR relaxation times and relaxation mechanisms from 1–100 MHz: dependence on tissue type, NMR frequency, temperature, species, excision, and age. Med Phys 1984;11(4):425–48.

[30] Norris DG. High field human imaging. J Magn Reson Imaging 2003;18(5):519–29.

[31] Stanisz GJ, Odrobina EE, Pun J, et al. T(1), T(2) relaxation and magnetization transfer in tissue at 3T. Magn Reson Med 2005;54(3):507–12.

[32] White LM, Buckwalter KA. Technical considerations: CT and MR imaging in the postoperative orthopedic patient. Semin Musculoskelet Radiol 2002;6(1):5–17.

[33] Collins CM, Liu W, Wang J, et al. Temperature and SAR calculations for a human head within volume and surface coils at 64 and 300 MHz. J Magn Reson Imaging 2004;19(5):650–6.

[34] Alsop DC. The sensitivity of low flip angle RARE imaging. Magn Reson Med 1997;37(2):176–84.

[35] Hennig J, Weigel M, Scheffler K. Multiecho sequences with variable refocusing flip angles: optimization of signal behavior using smooth transitions between pseudo steady states (TRAPS). Magn Reson Med 2003;49(3):527–35.

[36] Hennig J, Weigel M, Scheffler K. Calculation of flip angles for echo trains with predefined amplitudes with the extended phase graph (EPG)-algorithm: principles and applications to hyperecho and TRAPS sequences. Magn Reson Med 2004;51(1):68–80.

[37] Hennig J, Scheffler K. Hyperechoes. Magn Reson Med 2001;46(1):6–12.

[38] Feinberg DA, Oshio K. GRASE (gradient- and spin-echo) MR imaging: a new fast clinical imaging technique. Radiology 1991;181(2):597–602.

[39] Fullerton GD, Cameron IL, Ord VA. Orientation of tendons in the magnetic field and its effect on T2 relaxation times. Radiology 1985;155(2):433–5.

[40] Schmid MR, Notzli HP, Zanetti M, et al. Cartilage lesions in the hip: diagnostic effectiveness of MR arthrography. Radiology 2003;226(2):382–6.

[41] Kassarjian A, Yoon LS, Belzile E, et al. Triad of MR arthrographic findings in patients with cam-type femoroacetabular impingement. Radiology 2005;236(2):588–92.

[42] Ito K, Leunig M, Ganz R. Histopathologic features of the acetabular labrum in femoroacetabular impingement. Clin Orthop Relat Res 2004; 429:262–71.

[43] Plotz GM, Brossmann J, von Knoch M, et al. Magnetic resonance arthrography of the acetabular labrum: value of radial reconstructions. Arch Orthop Trauma Surg 2001;121(8):450–7.

[44] Mintz DN, Hooper T, Connell D, et al. Magnetic resonance imaging of the hip: detection of labral and chondral abnormalities using noncontrast imaging. Arthroscopy 2005;21(4):385–93.

[45] Nishii T, Tanaka H, Nakanishi K, et al. Fat-suppressed 3D spoiled gradient-echo MRI and MDCT arthrography of articular cartilage in patients with hip dysplasia. AJR Am J Roentgenol 2005;185(2):379–85.

[46] Keeney JA, Peelle MW, Jackson J, et al. Magnetic resonance arthrography versus arthroscopy in the evaluation of articular hip pathology. Clin Orthop Relat Res 2004;(429):163–9.

[47] Gold GE, Suh B, Sawyer-Glover A, et al. Musculoskeletal MRI at 3.0 T: initial clinical experience. AJR Am J Roentgenol 2004;183(5):1479–86.

[48] Gold GE, Han E, Stainsby J, et al. Musculoskeletal MRI at 3.0 T: relaxation times and image contrast. AJR Am J Roentgenol 2004;183(2):343–51.

[49] Fischbach F, Bruhn H, Unterhauser F, et al. Magnetic resonance imaging of hyaline cartilage defects at 1.5T and 3.0T: comparison of medium T2-weighted fast spin echo, T1-weighted two-dimensional and three-dimensional gradient echo pulse sequences. Acta Radiol 2005;46(1): 67–73.

[50] Hargreaves BA, Gold GE, Beaulieu CF, et al. Comparison of new sequences for high-resolution cartilage imaging. Magn Reson Med 2003; 49(4):700–9.

[51] Gold GE, Fuller SE, Hargreaves BA, et al. Driven equilibrium magnetic resonance imaging of articular cartilage: initial clinical experience. J Magn Reson Imaging 2005;21(4):476–81.

[52] Schmid MR, Pfirrmann CW, Koch P, et al. Imaging of patellar cartilage with a 2D multiple-echo data image combination sequence. AJR Am J Roentgenol 2005;184(6):1744–8.

[53] Masi JN, Sell CA, Phan C, et al. Cartilage MR imaging at 3.0 versus that at 1.5 T: preliminary results in a porcine model. Radiology 2005; 236(1):140–50.

[54] Schibany N, Ba-Ssalamah A, Marlovits S, et al. Impact of high field (3.0 T) magnetic resonance imaging on diagnosis of osteochondral defects in the ankle joint. Eur J Radiol 2005;55(2): 283–8.

[55] Schroder RJ, Fischbach F, Unterhauser FN, et al. [Value of various MR sequences using 1.5 and 3.0 Tesla in analyzing cartilaginous defects of the patella in an animal model]. Rofo 2004; 176(11):1667–75.

[56] Dardzinski BJ, Schmithorst VJ, Holland SK, et al. MR imaging of murine arthritis using ultrasmall superparamagnetic iron oxide particles. Magn Reson Imaging 2001;19(9):1209–16.

[57] Mosher TJ. Imaging of rheumatoid arthritis: can MR imaging be used to monitor cellular response of disease? Radiology 2004;233(1):1–2.

[58] Lutz AM, Seemayer C, et al. Detection of synovial macrophages in an experimental rabbit model of antigen-induced arthritis: ultrasmall superparamagnetic iron oxide-enhanced MR imaging. Radiology 2004;233(1):149–57.

[59] Mosher TJ, Dardzinski BJ. Cartilage MRI T2 relaxation time mapping: overview and applications. Semin Musculoskelet Radiol 2004;8(4): 355–68.

[60] Burstein D, Velyvis J, Scott KT, et al. Protocol issues for delayed Gd(DTPA)(2-)-enhanced MRI (dGEMRIC) for clinical evaluation of articular cartilage. Magn Reson Med 2001;45(1):36–41.

[61] Tiderius CJ, Svensson J, Leander P, et al. dGEMRIC (delayed gadolinium-enhanced MRI of cartilage) indicates adaptive capacity of human knee cartilage. Magn Reson Med 2004;51(2):286–90.

[62] de Bazelaire CM, Duhamel GD, Rofsky NM, et al. MR imaging relaxation times of abdominal and pelvic tissues measured in vivo at 3.0 T: preliminary results. Radiology 2004;230(3):652–9.

MAGNETIC RESONANCE IMAGING CLINICS

Magn Reson Imaging Clin N Am (2006) 77–88

3T MR Imaging of the Brain

Mark C. DeLano MD*, Charles Fisher

- T1-weighted imaging
  T1 prolongation at 3T
  The role of the T1-weighted sequence
  Standing wave effects
  Pulse sequence options
  Conventional and fast spin echo
  Inversion-prepared sequences
- Gradient echo susceptibility (T2*) imaging
- T2-weighted imaging
- T2–fluid-attenuated inversion recovery imaging
- Diffusion-weighted imaging
- Orbit and skull base
- MR angiography
- Summary
- References

MR imaging devices that operate at very high field strengths (up to 4 T) received U.S. Food and Drug Administration clearance in 1998, and clinical 3T units were approved in 2001. Since that time the number of 3T sites and clinical applications for 3T continue to increase. The attraction to 3T is the theoretic doubling of signal without increasing the scan time that is associated with signal averaging; however, the increase in field strength is responsible for some of the primary limitations of this method to achieve a greater signal-to-noise ratio (SNR). Doubling the field requires doubling of the spin resonance frequency when compared with 1.5T. Specifically, this results in twice the energy deposition, which causes potential problems with limits in individual specific absorption rates (SARs), and twice the chemical shift misregistration.

Although most of the challenges that initially limited dissemination and adoption of 3T MR devices have been addressed by several approaches, the full potential of the added value of very high field is dependent on continued software and hardware development and the choices that are made in protocol implementation. As with the transitions between low-field open scanners and 1.5T

instruments, proper field-specific parameter selection remains important for the establishment of clinical protocols. Each pulse sequence requires field-specific modifications. This article discusses the issues of 3T clinical protocol development and implementation for brain imaging, and demonstrates methods to achieve the greatest potential of higher field strength systems.

An additional observation also is relevant given the multiple organ systems that are discussed in this issue. There is little tolerance for variation in normal image contrast features in neuroimaging because the reliance on the expected gray white contrast features of a sequence for anatomic assessment and delineation of pathology. Therefore, increased awareness of the contrast mechanisms at 3T is helpful in avoiding interpretive pitfalls [1].

T1-weighted imaging

T1 prolongation at 3T

The initial response to clinical 3T brain imaging was less than enthusiastic, primarily because of the low gray-to-white matter contrast in spin-echo T1 sequences [2]. The increased longitudinal relaxation

Department of Radiology, Michigan State University, 184 Radiology Building, East Lansing, MI 48824, USA
*Corresponding author.
E-mail address: mcd@rad.msu.edu (M.C. DeLano).

1064-9689/06/\$ – see front matter © 2006 Elsevier Inc. All rights reserved.
mri.theclinics.com

doi:10.1016/j.mric.2006.01.004

times of tissue at 3T result in the poor differentiation of gray and white matter. Although there is some variation in the literature, the T1 of white matter is 884 milliseconds at 1.5T, which is prolonged to 1084 milliseconds at 3T. Gray matter has a T1 of 1124 milliseconds at 1.5T and 1820 milliseconds at 3T [3–7]. Using a standard repetition time of 500 milliseconds for T1-weighted imaging results in convergence of gray and white matter signal intensities and tissue saturation effects that contribute to the poor gray and white matter differentiation.

The role of the T1-weighted sequence

There are many sequences available to acquire T1-weighted images of the brain; each has positive and negative attributes. Choice of approach requires a defined clinical role for the T1 sequence. When the primary concern is the delineation of anatomy to identify a migrational abnormality, one needs obvious gray–white differentiation. If the indication for the examination mandates the identification of enhancement, the need for intrinsic tissue contrast is minimal and could compromise the capacity to identify an enhancing lesion by diminishing lesion to background contrast. White matter is hyperintense on T1-weighted images before contrast, particularly on inversion-prepared T1-weighted sequences compared with spin echo (SE) or fast spin echo (FSE) images. Saturation of nonenhancing background tissue improves the detection of contrast enhancement. This has fueled interest in magnetization transfer phenomena since Wolff and Balaban's [8] description of the process in 1989. Therefore, it is unclear why there has been such focus on gray–white contrast in T1-weighted imaging, aside from a general resistance to change and an aesthetic gravitation to images with more contrast. It is arguable that the most important function of the T1 sequence is the identification of abnormal regions of contrast accumulation. The need to identify subtle migrational abnormalities is real, but is far less common in general practice than the need to identify a cerebral metastasis or demyelinating lesion. Additionally, the information regarding gray–white differentiation is readily available from quality T2-weighted images. These can be gray scale inverted to give the impression of T1 weighting if desired, but obviously the usefulness simply would be limited to display preference (Figs. 1 and 2).

Standing wave effects

Before discussing the relative attributes of these pulse sequences, the concept of standing wave effects, or so-called "dielectric resonance effects," needs to be introduced. Standing wave effects

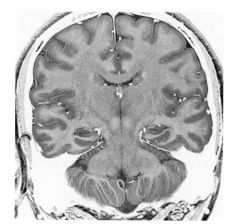

Figure 1 Coronal FSE T2-weighted image demonstrates excellent gray–white differentiation. Note the cytoarchitectural detail of the hippocampus (TR 3200 milliseconds, TE 79.4 milliseconds, ETL 16, NEX 4, matrix 512 × 224, FOV 16 cm, 3-mm interleaved slices, 6:12).

contribute, in general, to image nonuniformity, and specifically, to problems with contrast in the brain. The wavelength of the radiofrequency (RF) energy that is used at 3T is in close proportion to the size of the head. This causes the generation of standing waves and constructive and destructive interference patterns that result in a heterogeneous signal in the brain. This is manifested as central hyperintensity of the deeper structures and relative hypointensity of the more superficial structures. This effect is present at all fields and on all sequences to varying degrees, but is accentuated at higher fields and is clearly evident with the use of quadrature coils on T1-weighted sequences. Fig. 3 demonstrates the impact of the standing wave effect on an axial FSE T1-weighted image that was generated with a quadrature head coil. The effect is balanced largely by using eight-channel phased-array head coils and the associated signal intensity uniformity correction algorithms that are used commonly in general clinical imaging. The advent of eight-channel coils has made this effect essentially negligible, but it is included here to provide added insight into the challenges that faced the early 3T users and the underlying issues of image contrast at 3T.

Pulse sequence options

The initial desire to seek out alternatives to conventional spin echo (CSE) was driven by poor gray–white contrast and difficulties with SAR management. The development of the phased-array coil and pulse sequence modifications largely has resolved these issues. Fig. 2 demonstrates the marked improvement in image quality, gray–white contrast, and the SNR that is generated by the eight-channel

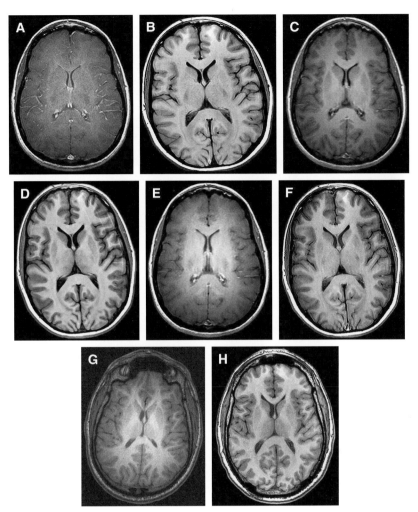

Figure 2 Marked improvement in image quality, gray–white contrast, and SNR is seen with the eight-channel coil (*B, D, F, H*) compared with the quadrature coil (*A, C, E, G*) using four different T1-weighted sequences. (*A, B*) Conventional spin echo (TR 700 milliseconds, TE 13 milliseconds, NEX 2, FOV 22 × 17 cm, matrix 384 × 192, 22 slices, 3:26). (*C, D*) T1 FLAIR (TR 3142 milliseconds, TE 9.9 milliseconds, TI 920, ETL 7, NEX 2, FOV 22 × 17 cm, matrix 384 × 192, 22 slices, 2:29). (*E, F*) FSE (TR 700 milliseconds, TE 10.1 milliseconds, ETL 2, NEX 2, FOV 22 cm, matrix 384 × 192, 28 slices, 3:25). (*G, H*) Inversion-prepared fast spoiled echo gradient (TR 9.1 milliseconds, TE 3.9 milliseconds, FA 20, NEX 1, IR prep 450, FOV 24 × 18 cm, matrix 352 × 224, 1.33 mm/120 locations, 5:41).

coil compared with the quadrature coil using four different T1-weighted sequences. CSE and FSE will be discussed together, and a discussion of inversion prepared sequence follows.

Conventional and fast spin echo

CSE T1-weighted imaging is SAR intensive, particularly on earlier scanner models, before improvements in pulse sequence design, and in the SAR calculation algorithms. The linear increase in signal intensity with increasing B0 (main static magnetic) field strength is associated with SAR increases that are proportional to the square of the B0 field strength, or resonance frequency. In response to the SAR demands of T1 weighting and the desire

for better contrast, the spin echo pulse sequence has been modified to improve both. Schmitz and colleagues [9] evaluated the role of flip angle in the modulation of gray–white contrast and SAR. Their rationale was that because the deposition of RF power is related to the square of excitation pulse at 90° and image contrast is suboptimal at 3T, both issues could be addressed by decreasing the flip angle of the 90° RF pulse (RF1). They showed a substantial effect of different flip angles on gray-to-white matter contrast in 3T imaging, with the best contrast-to-noise ratio (CNR) at the lowest flip angle of 50°. There were associated decreases in SAR and SNR. Schmitz and colleagues [9] performed this study using a quadrature coil. The authors repeated their

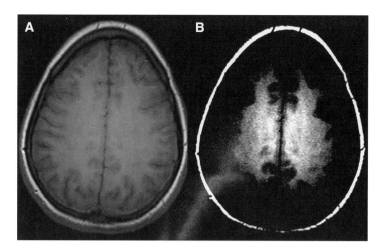

Figure 3 The impact of the standing wave effect on an axial FSE T1-weighted image generated with a quadrature head coil (TR 700 milliseconds, TE 10.1 milliseconds, ETL 2, FOV 23 cm, matrix 320 × 192. (*A*) Standard window width and level. (*B*) Narrow window width accentuates the inhomogeneity of the image and central hyperintensity.

experiment by using an eight-channel coil, and demonstrated a similar phenomenon (Fig. 4). Increased differentiation between gray and white matter is shown (see Fig. 4A), which was obtained by using a 50° flip angle instead of 90° (see Fig. 4B). Decreased SNR and SAR also were seen in the authors' examples using a 50° flip angle. The degree of SNR reduction that the authors observed was more than 40%, which severely reduced the benefit of doubling the field strength. The authors have opted to maintain their RF1 flip angle at 90° degrees. The currently implemented version of the authors' T1 spin echo protocol uses a reduced refocusing pulse (RF2) of 120° instead of 180°, which addresses the need for SAR reduction. There is an effect on image contrast because of the reduction in RF2, which contributes to improved contrast and also reduces the SNR. Fig. 5 demonstrates the improvement in contrast in an FSE T1-weighted image by the reduction of RF2 to 120° and by leaving RF1 unchanged (90°). A similar effect is observed with CSE.

The authors have found that the image quality of CSE is superior to FSE for T1 weighting, primarily because it provides a balance between the competing interests of gray–white contrast generation and SNR, without the concern for image blurring. The imaging times are comparable because of the need to perform interleaved acquisitions for FSE as a result of cross-talk–related signal loss on alternating images. Although FSE blur can be minimized with short echo train lengths, increased receiver bandwidth to minimize echo spacing, and the use of tailored RF pulses, there is typically more blur in the FSE image than that achieved with CSE. Compared with SE sequences that are acquired with the same parameters, there is an attendant loss of signal that is proportionate to the echo train length for short echo time (TE) sequences. Interleaving could allow shorter repetition times (TRs); however, this is counterproductive in terms of the signal loss that is due to the saturation effects that are associated with the longer T1 of tissues.

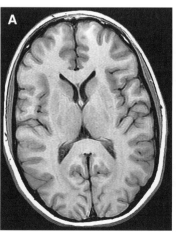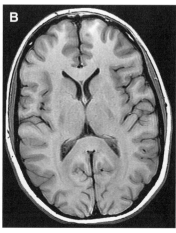

Figure 4 Reducing the flip angle (RF1) on CSE T1-weighted images (TR 700 milliseconds, TE 13 milliseconds, NEX 2) improves gray–white contrast and results in diminished SAR and SNR. (*A*) Flip angle 50°. Better visualization of the putamina and internal lamina but decreased SNR (13 vs. 23), decreased estimated SAR (1.83 vs. 2.00 W/kg), and decreased peak SAR (3.66 vs. 4.00 W/kg). (*B*) Flip angle 90°.

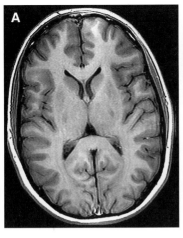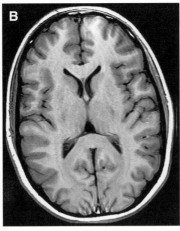

Figure 5 Reducing the flip angle (RF2) on FSE T1-weighted images (TR 700 milliseconds, TE 10.1 milliseconds, NEX 2, ETL 2, interleaved 5-mm slices) improves gray–white contrast and results in diminished SAR and SNR. (A) Refocusing pulse flip angle 120°. Better gray–white differentiation is noted and there is decreased SNR (13 vs. 20), decreased estimated SAR (0.86 vs. 1.40 W/kg), and decreased peak SAR (1.72 vs. 2.80 W/kg). (B) Refocusing pulse flip angle 180°.

A compelling alternative view regarding the use of shorter TR times for contrast MR imaging was presented by Krautmacher and colleagues [10]. They found surprising results in their recent study that compared single- and half-dose contrast at 3T with single-dose contrast at 1.5T. The CNR was 2.8-fold greater when using single-dose contrast at 3T, than when using single-dose contrast at 1.5T. The explanation lies in the doubling that is expected to occur as a result of field change, combined with the benefit of using the same TR as that used at 1.5T (ie, 500 milliseconds). Because the brain has longer tissue T1 relaxation times at 3T, the use of the same TR as at 1.5T yields stronger T1 weighting. This manifests as lower signal in nonenhancing tissue than is predicted by the change in field strength alone, and is analogous to a saturation effect. Because enhancing tissues have short T1 relaxation times they relax nearly completely after each TR, even with a short TR of 500 milliseconds. This results in a twofold increase in signal for the enhancing tissues. The combined effect of diminished background signal (less than two times predicted) and doubling of the lesion signal yields a greater than twofold increase of lesion–brain CNR at 3T. Administration of half-dose contrast at 3T resulted in 1.3 times the CNR that was observed at 1.5T. The clinical translation of the increased signal that is afforded by the investment in 3T is the opportunity to reduce contrast dose by half, while maintaining CNR that is greater than that usually observed at 1.5T.

Magnetization transfer (MT) contrast is an important contrast determinant in multislice T1-weighted hybrid RARE (rapid acquisition with relaxation enhancement) sequences [6,11,12]. This effect may improve lesion conspicuity after contrast administration [8,13–15]. The differential signal between gray and white matter is diminished by MT effects that are inherent in the FSE sequences. The effect is greater at 3T compared with 1.5T [6], and reduces MT ratios (MTR) by 2% to 10% because of the T1 prolongation effects on the MTR measurement [5,16]. The use of MT pulses for T1-weighted imaging of the brain is SAR intensive and is not performed routinely. The opportunity to do so may arise as new pulse sequences are developed that apply the MT pulse only during the acquisition of the central lines of k-space, as has been reported for MR angiography (MRA). This selective application of the MT pulse has the important effect of altering contrast while limiting the SAR.

Inversion-prepared sequences

Inversion-prepared sequences also have been advocated for T1 weighting because the resultant gray–white contrast is superior to other methods. T1 FLAIR (fluid-attenuated inversion recovery) and inversion-prepared 3D fast spoiled gradient echo (FSPGR) sequences exhibit robust gray–white contrast. T1 FLAIR sequences use an FSE readout with diminished RF2 to help manage SAR. The 3D FSPGR that is used by the authors is inversion prepared, and is the least SAR intensive of the four methods of T1 weighting. The resulting images from both show impressive gray–white contrast features (see Fig. 2). Image quality is affected by SNR, CNR, and lesion-to-background contrast. Obviously, SNR and lesion conspicuity, including the capacity to demonstrate contrast enhancement, need to be considered. A common feature of both inversion-prepared sequences is that lesions that show T2 hyperintensity are hypointense on these T1-weighted sequences more commonly than they are on spin echo or FSE sequences. This may have importance in the appearance of enhancing lesions that are markedly hypointense on precontrast T1-weighted images where the additive effect of precontrast hypointensity and postcontrast hyperintensity

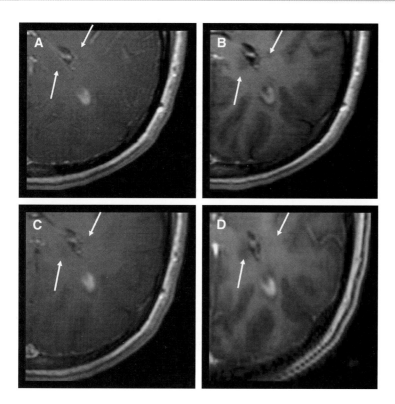

Figure 6 Differential lesion-to-background contrast using four different T1-weighted sequences. CSE (*A*), T1 FLAIR (*B*), FSE (*C*), and 3D FSPGR (*D*). Nonenhancing lesions (*arrows*) are more hypointense on inversion-prepared sequences (*B, D*). Enhancing lesions vary in conspicuity relative to background white matter signal intensity.

result in isointensity to surrounding normal tissues. Melhem and colleagues [17] showed that the conspicuity and number of contrast-enhancing lesions are greater for CSE sequences than for T1 FLAIR sequences. Again, the issue of competing desires for anatomically appealing gray–white contrast and for diagnostically useful images that demonstrate enhancing pathology is raised. In the authors' experience this issue is primarily that of the capacity to detect a small area of enhancement, such as that seen in multiple sclerosis or in a small solitary metastatic deposit (Fig. 6). The contrast features of enhancing and nonenhancing lesions vary depending on the lesion and the sequence that is used for T1 weighting. In a small series of patients that was seen in the authors' center, the SNR and CNR were greatest for the FSE sequence, which offers the potential for improved detection of enhancing lesions. Contrast enhancement and lesion-to-background contrast for these patients are shown in Table 1.

Although the 3D FSPGR sequence is the longest of the scans, and therefore, is more motion sensitive, the images can be reformatted into any plane and have excellent gray–white differentiation. Although there was initial concern that these gradient echo images would have excessive distortion because of susceptibility artifacts, this has not been a significant issue in practice.

Gradient echo susceptibility (T2*) imaging

Detection of spontaneous or posttraumatic hemorrhage by MR imaging is facilitated by the use of a dedicated T2* or susceptibility sequence. The sequence, as implemented by the authors, is less than

Table 1: Enhancing lesion conspicuity in multiple sclerosis using four pulse sequences to demonstrate differential contrast features, signal-to-noise ratio, and scan time

T1 sequence	SI lesion postcontrast	SI normal white matter	Lesion/background contrast	SNR	Scan time
FSE	379	251	1.51	46	3:18
SE	407	290	1.4	33	4:26
FSPGR	653	502	1.3	27	5:43
T1 FLAIR	324	310	1.04	42	3:57

Abbreviation: SI, signal intensity.

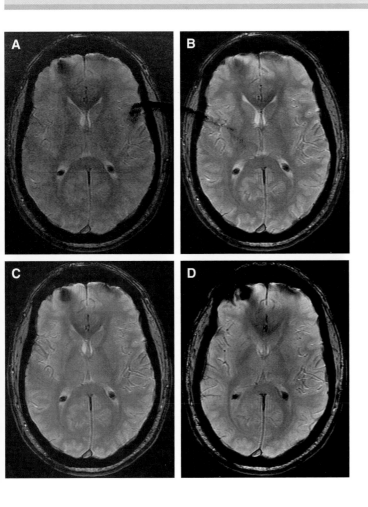

Figure 7 Susceptibility (T2*)-weighted images demonstrate the effect of flip angle modulation on the degree of magnetic susceptibility while TE is fixed at 20 milliseconds (TR 500 milliseconds for all). (*A*) 5° flip angle with severe loss of signal, (*B*) 15° flip angle, (*C*) 20° flip angle, (*D*) 40° flip angle. Increasing flip angle increases the susceptibility weighting. At 3T, the author's clinical sequence uses a 15° flip angle with a TE of 20 milliseconds.

2 minutes and often adds substantively to the capacity to identify foci of blood products or calcification. This has become increasingly important with the use of long echo train length FSE T2 sequences.

Optimization of the sequence required modification of the 1.5T protocol with decreased TE and flip angle for the 3T protocol (Figs. 7 and 8). Decreasing the flip angle and TE diminish the T2* sensitivity. These changes were necessary to reduce the skull base and paranasal sinus region artifacts. Occult blood products that are associated with hypertensive hemorrhages, occult vascular malformations, or other vascular disorders are much more conspicuous on the T2* sequence than on the FSE T2 sequence that is obtained at the same time (Fig. 9).

Increased sensitivity to local field alterations offers a unique opportunity to improve upon functional MR (fMR) imaging using blood oxygen level–dependent contrast. There is doubling of the fMR imaging signal at 3T compared with 1.5T. This can lead to improved accuracy in detecting regions of activation with greater confidence, identify sites of activation not otherwise noted, or increase

spatial resolution. Increasing spatial resolution can generate more fMR imaging signal by diminishing the partial volume averaging effect that is caused by using a larger region of interest [18–20].

T2-weighted imaging

T2 shortening at 3T in the brain is negligible. Some of the most dramatic improvement in image quality that is due to increased field strength is seen in T2-weighted imaging of the brain. Contrary to the initial response to T1-weighted imaging at 3T, much enthusiasm has been generated for T2 image quality. The T2 relaxation times of tissue at 3T do not result in significant changes in the contrast between gray and white matter. The T2 of white matter is 72 milliseconds at 1.5T and 69 milliseconds at 3T, whereas the T2 of gray matter is 95 milliseconds at 1.5T and 99 milliseconds at 3T [4,6,21]. T2-weighted imaging results in robust gray and white matter differentiation and excellent delineation of pathology. The adaptation of the FSE sequences to the 3T system required careful modifications to the pulse sequences, including the use of reduced

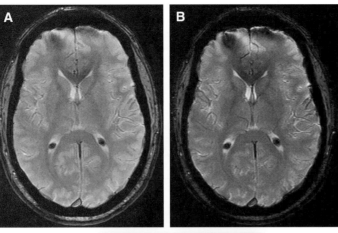

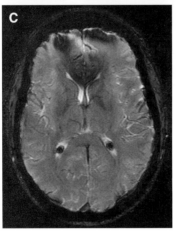

Figure 8 Susceptibility (T2*)-weighted images demonstrate the effect of TE modulation on the degree of magnetic susceptibility while flip angle is fixed at 15° (TR 500 milliseconds for all). (*A*) TE 20 milliseconds, (*B*) TE 30 milliseconds, (*C*) TE 40 milliseconds. Increasing TE increases the susceptibility weighting. At 3T, the author's clinical sequence uses a 15° flip angle with a TE of 20 milliseconds.

and tailored RF2 (180°). The widespread acceptance of FSE T2 and FLAIR sequences in clinical practice at 3T is supported further by evolving techniques that are not sensitive to motion, such as periodically rotated overlapping parallel lines with enhanced reconstruction (PROPELLER) [22–24]. The motion insensitivity of the PROPELLER method originates in the collection of data in concentric rectangular strips that are rotated about the k-space origin. There is oversampling of the central region of k-space, which allows one to correct spatial inconsistencies in position, rotation, and phase between strips. Therefore, one can reject data based on a correlation measure that indicates through-

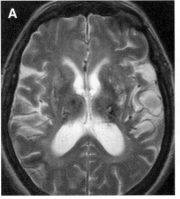

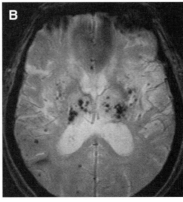

Figure 9 FSE T2 (*A*) and susceptibility (T2*)-weighted images (*B*) demonstrate the marked increase in degree of sensitivity to magnetic susceptibility with the gradient echo technique. (*A*) TR 3550 milliseconds, TE 102 milliseconds, ETL 20. (*B*) 3T clinical sequence using a 15° flip angle and a TE of 20 milliseconds reveals many additional foci of chronic hemorrhage.

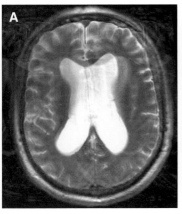

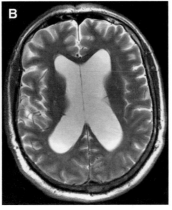

Figure 10 3T PROPELLER T2 sequence in patient who has Parkinson's disease. (*A*) Motion severely degrades image quality with standard FSE T2 sequence. (*B*) PROPELLER T2-weighted image reduces artifact without sedation.

plane motion, and further decreases motion artifacts through an averaging effect for low spatial frequencies. The "spraying" of artifacts, such as pulsatility artifacts, that normally are propagated in the phase-encoding direction also improves image quality (Fig. 10).

T2–fluid-attenuated inversion recovery imaging

Optimizing image contrast and lesion conspicuity are the primary challenges of the T2-FLAIR sequence (Fig. 11). There is improved image contrast with increasing TE and TR. Echo time is controlled primarily by echo train length and the choice of receiver bandwidth. Increasing the echo train length has the capacity to diminish lesion conspicuity through generation of FSE blur, but this does not seem to be the case with PROPELLER, possibly because of the oversampling of central k-space. Inversion time is dependent on the other parameters that are selected, but is slightly longer at 3T compared with 1.5T (Fig. 12). The importance of TE and TR in image contrast outcome is crucial at 3T. There is a central hyperintensity to normal white matter

that can reduce CNR when using 1.5T parameters on a 3T scanner for T2-FLAIR. 3D FLAIR is another alternative that has potential usefulness in the diagnostic armamentarium, particularly for thin section multiplanar reconstructions in the evaluation of demyelinating disease.

Diffusion-weighted imaging

The capacity to perform single-shot echo planar diffusion-weighted imaging (DWI) at 3T is boosted by additional signal that allows for increased resolution. Increased susceptibility artifacts at 3T were problematic early on. The image quality has improved markedly, primarily because of the introduction of the eight-channel coil. This coil allowed for parallel imaging and marked reduction of the echo time from 98 milliseconds to 60 milliseconds at a b value of 1000 s/mm^2 (Fig. 13). The introduction of PROPELLER DWI was the other major influence on how DWI is performed. Although there is no inherent correction of motion with this technique, the major contribution is the capacity to eliminate susceptibility artifact at the skull base, which is a particularly vexing problem at 3T.

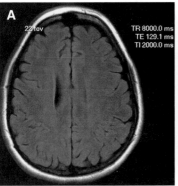

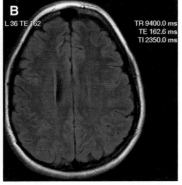

Figure 11 PROPELLER FLAIR images. Improved gray–white differentiation with increasing TR, echo train, and TE. (*A*) TR 8000 milliseconds, TE 129 milliseconds, TI 2000, ETL 32. (*B*) TR 9400 milliseconds, TE 163 milliseconds, TI 2350, ETL 36.

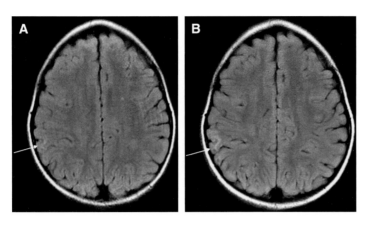

Figure 12 PROPELLER FLAIR image of unsedated 6-year-old patient who sustained head trauma (*A*) compared with standard FSE FLAIR image (*B*). Small cortical right frontoparietal lobe contusion (*arrow*) is more conspicuous on the PROPELLER image because of motion suppression.

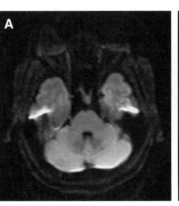
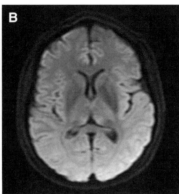

Figure 13 Diffusion-weighted imaging at 3T. (*A*) Skull base–related artifacts are reduced using parallel imaging, which results in reduced TE and fewer phase-encoding steps. (*B*) Note diminished signal intensity of the basal ganglia that is due to iron deposition and T2* signal loss. TR 8000 milliseconds, TE 60.8 milliseconds, b-value 1000.

Orbit and skull base

Much of the initial concern that susceptibility artifacts and off resonance effects would interfere with fat suppression were ill founded. There is a relative ease of suppression of fat at 3T, because of the increased chemical shift between water and fat. The clinical results are remarkable for uniform fat saturation and excellent contrast enhancement. Higher receiver bandwidth settings are needed to reduce chemical shift artifact on the nonfat-suppressed sequences because of the abundant fat–soft tissue interfaces. The increase in receiver bandwidth also allows for reduced echo spacing and TE values, which help to minimize skull base–associated susceptibility artifacts (Figs. 14 and 15).

MR angiography

3T MRA benefits from several key phenomena. The theoretic SNR of 3T is twice that of 1.5T; this offers the opportunity to increase the spatial resolution or to shorten scan times by up to a factor of four. MRA benefits from the longer T1s of tissues at 3T—which are 20% to 40% longer than at 1.5T—and provides

better background suppression, additional inflow enhancement, and improved CNR. MT normally would be considered to be SAR prohibitive at 3T, but a novel pulse sequence design has overcome this challenge by applying the SAR-intensive MT pulse to only the center of k-space. The appropriate choice of imaging parameters can minimize artifacts and exploit T1 prolongation at higher fields

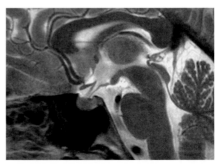

Figure 14 Negligible susceptibility artifact about the skull base on sagittal FSE T2-weighted image. TR 3200 milliseconds, TE 102 milliseconds, ETL 16, NEX 2.

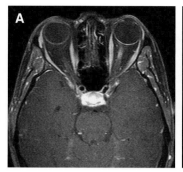
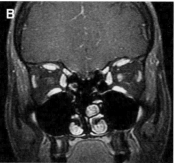

Figure 15 Uniform fat saturation in the orbits in the axial (*A*) and coronal (*B*) planes in a patient who has multiple sclerosis and left optic neuritis. Excellent delineation of abnormal enhancement.

for better quality MRA. As with 1.5T MRA, 3T MRA requires proper balancing of the choice of receiver bandwidth and echo time minimization (32 kHz, TE 2–3 milliseconds), so that susceptibility artifacts and complex flow-related signal loss are minimized. As the quality of MRA continues to improve the potential to replace conventional diagnostic angiography grows; this begs the question "is vasculitis an MRA diagnosis" (Fig. 16)? Improved quality of imaging of cerebral aneurysms has been reported at 3T compared with at 1.5T [25,26].

The availability of scanners that are capable of parallel imaging, together with the increasing availability of multichannel coils, is coincident with the arrival of these very high field scanners. Early results with using these combined advancements for intracranial MRA yielded spatial resolution that exceeded invasive digital subtraction angiography (DSA) and provided breathtaking visualization of small arteries, such as the lenticulostriate vasculature. The efficiency of the parallel imaging approach also complements the quality of time-resolved MRA techniques and increases the temporal resolution proportionately to the acceleration factor.

Summary

The advent of very high field clinical scanners that operate at 3T is taking structural and functional imaging to new levels and is reinvigorating clinical spectroscopy, fMR imaging, and noncontrast-enhanced methods of MRA. Most of the challenges that are related to 3T imaging have been addressed to facilitate routine clinical imaging. An awareness of the complexities that underlie the solutions to these challenges is important to the continued improvements to the 3T platform so that its maximal potential can be reached.

The development of the multichannel-head coils and the improvement in the design of body coils, concurrently with the development of multichannel capabilities that enable parallel imaging, have benefited all field platforms. Perhaps the added value of parallel imaging has been greatest at 3T where the additional signal can be exploited. The definition of very high field is a moving target, and may be well on its way to 7.0 T, although in terms of the current clinical state of the art, 3T is our current reference.

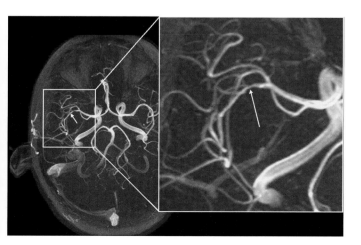

Figure 16 High-resolution unenhanced 3D time-of-flight MRA of the intracranial circulation. Atherosclerotic narrowing in the M3 portion of the right middle cerebral artery (*arrow*). TR 30 milliseconds, TE 3.4 milliseconds, FOV 22 × 16.5 cm, 512 × 256 matrix zero-filled to 1024, 31.25 kHz receiver bandwidth.

References

[1] Schmitz BL, Aschoff AJ, Hoffmann MH, et al. Advantages and pitfalls in 3T MR brain imaging: a pictorial review. AJNR Am J Neuroradiol 2005; 26:2229–37.

[2] Ross JS. The high-field-strength curmudgeon. AJNR Am J Neuroradiol 2004;25:168–9.

[3] Ethofer T, Mader I, Seeger U, et al. Comparison of longitudinal metabolite relaxation times in different regions of the human brain at 1.5 and 3 Tesla. Magn Reson Med 2003;50:1296–301.

[4] Hendrick RE. Image contrast and noise. In: Stark DD, Bradley WG, editors. Magnetic resonance imaging, vol. 1. 3rd edition. St. Louis (MO): Mosby; 1999. p. 43–67.

[5] Sled JG, Pike GB. Quantitative imaging of magnetization transfer exchange and relaxation properties in vivo using MRI. Magn Reson Med 2001; 46:923–31.

[6] Stanisz GJ, Odrobina EE, Pun J, et al. T1, T2 relaxation and magnetization transfer in tissue at 3T. Magn Reson Med 2005;54:507–12.

[7] Wansapura JP, Holland SK, Dunn RS, et al. NMR relaxation times in the human brain at 3.0 Tesla. J Magn Reson Imaging 1999;9:531–8.

[8] Wolff SD, Balaban RS. Magnetization transfer contrast (MTC) and tissue water proton relaxation in vivo. Magn Reson Med 1989;10:135–44.

[9] Schmitz BL, Gron G, Brausewetter F, et al. Enhancing gray-to-white matter contrast in 3T T1 spin-echo brain scans by optimizing flip angle. AJNR Am J Neuroradiol 2005;26:2000–4.

[10] Krautmacher C, Willinek WA, Tschampa HJ, et al. Brain tumors: full- and half-dose contrast-enhanced MR imaging at 3.0 T compared with 1.5 T—initial experience. Radiology 2005; 237:1014–9.

[11] Melhem ER, Jara H, Yucel EK. Multislice T1-weighted hybrid RARE in CNS imaging: assessment of magnetization transfer effects and artifacts. J Magn Reson Imaging 1996;6:903–8.

[12] Melki PS, Mulkern RV. Magnetization transfer effects in multislice RARE sequences. Magn Reson Med 1992;24:189–95.

[13] Elster AD, King JC, Mathews VP, et al. Cranial tissues: appearance at gadolinium-enhanced and nonenhanced MR imaging with magnetization transfer contrast. Radiology 1994;190:541–6.

[14] Elster AD, Mathews VP, King JC, et al. Improved detection of gadolinium enhancement using magnetization transfer imaging. Neuroimaging Clin N Am 1994;4:185–92.

[15] Wolff SD, Balaban RS. Magnetization transfer imaging: practical aspects and clinical applications. Radiology 1994;192:593–9.

[16] Duvvuri U, Roberts DA, Leigh JS, et al. Magnetization transfer imaging of the brain: a quantitative comparison of results obtained at 1.5 and 4.0 T. J Magn Reson Imaging 1999;10:527–32.

[17] Hoenig K, Kuhl CK, Scheef L. Functional 3.0-T MR assessment of higher cognitive function: are there advantages over 1.5-T imaging? Radiology 2005;234:860–8.

[18] Thulborn KR. Clinical rationale for very-high-field (3.0 Tesla) functional magnetic resonance imaging. Top Magn Reson Imaging 1999; 10:37–50.

[19] Melhem ER, Bert RJ, Walker RE. Usefulness of optimized gadolinium-enhanced fast fluid-attenuated inversion recovery MR imaging in revealing lesions of the brain. AJR Am J Roentgenol 1998;171:803–7.

[20] Thulborn KR. Why neuroradiologists should consider very-high-field magnets for clinical applications of functional magnetic resonance imaging. Top Magn Reson Imaging 1999;10:1–2.

[21] Briellmann RS, Jackson GD, Pell GS, et al. Structural abnormalities remote from the seizure focus: a study using T2 relaxometry at 3 T. Neurology 2004;63:2303–8.

[22] Forbes KP, Pipe JG, Bird CR, et al. PROPELLER MRI: clinical testing of a novel technique for quantification and compensation of head motion. J Magn Reson Imaging 2001;14:215–22.

[23] Forbes KP, Pipe JG, Karis JP, et al. Improved image quality and detection of acute cerebral infarction with PROPELLER diffusion-weighted MR imaging. Radiology 2002;225:551–5.

[24] Pipe JG. Motion correction with PROPELLER MRI: application to head motion and free-breathing cardiac imaging. Magn Reson Med 1999; 42:963–9.

[25] Gibbs GF, Huston J III, Bernstein MA, et al. 3.0-Tesla MR angiography of intracranial aneurysms: comparison of time-of-flight and contrast-enhanced techniques. J Magn Reson Imaging 2005;21:97–102.

[26] Gibbs GF, Huston J III, Bernstein MA, et al. Improved image quality of intracranial aneurysms: 3.0-T versus 1.5 T time-of-flight MR angiography. AJNR Am J Neuroradiol 2004;25:84–7.

ELSEVIER
SAUNDERS

MAGNETIC
RESONANCE
IMAGING CLINICS

Magn Reson Imaging Clin N Am (2006) 89–95

Head and Neck Imaging at 3T

Nafi Aygun MD*, S. James Zinreich MD

- Summary
- References

In the past decades significant advances in imaging with 1.5T units have benefited head and neck imaging. It is hoped that the 3T units, now commercially available, will provide an exponential advance in the evaluation of this body part. This article aims to justify our expectations based on physical principles. A discussion of the advantages and disadvantages of head and neck imaging at 3T in our experience and those of others is provided.

The clear advantage of the 3T magnets is the higher signal-to-noise ratio (SNR), which provides additional spatial resolution or time. In evaluation of the head and neck region, high-resolution imaging is needed because of the small size of many of the anatomic and pathologic structures. Decreasing total scanning time also is important, particularly in patients who have diseases of the head and neck region and who cannot tolerate long image acquisitions because of airway or swallowing difficulties.

Major challenges that come with the "3T package" include increased chemical shift and susceptibility artifacts. These are particularly troublesome in head and neck imaging because the intimate presence of air, bone, and acute changes in tissue bulk result in locoregional field distortions that are proportional to the static magnetic field, and thus, are worsened at 3T.

In clinical practice, one of the immediate benefits of 3T magnets was observed in the area of T2-weighted (T2W) imaging. T2W imaging using rapid acquisition with relaxation enhancement (RARE; aka fast spin echo or turbo spin echo) sequence, high matrix sizes (eg, 512×512), and thinner slices provide high spatial resolution (Figs. 1–4). RARE sequence uses a radiofrequency (RF) excitation pulse followed by a train of refocusing pulses that suppress field inhomogeneities and susceptibility effects that are created by air, bone, and sharp changes in tissue contour in the head and neck. Fat suppression—an absolute necessity in evaluation of the skull base and neck—is achieved using frequency-selective techniques, and counteracts with increased chemical shift, a welcome side benefit.

Challenges include decreased SNR from increased matrix size and thinner slices. In addition, image blurring that compromises spatial resolution—a problem for T2W RARE sequences with long echo trains—increases in high field imaging because of shortened T2. The degree of change in T2 with increasing field is tissue dependent as described recently by de Bazelaire and colleagues [1]. With high performance gradient capability, one can reduce echo spacing to minimize the signal loss that is associated with shortening of T2. Maintaining echo train lengths (ETLs) at less than 32 keeps image blurring at acceptable levels. Increased chemical shift and susceptibility artifacts that are due to higher field may hinder the diagnostic quality of the study (Fig. 5). These can be mitigated by increasing bandwidth and ETL; however, this approach can have deleterious effects on SNR and image blurring.

The Russell H. Morgan Department of Radiology and Radiological Sciences, The Johns Hopkins Medical Institution, 600 North Wolfe Street/Phipps B-126-A, Baltimore, MD 21287, USA
*Corresponding author.
E-mail address: naygun1@jhmi.edu (N. Aygun).

doi:10.1016/j.mric.2006.01.002

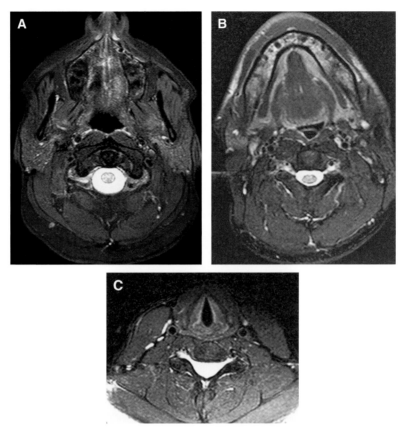

Figure 1 Axial T2W images through the nasopharynx (*A*), floor of the mouth (*B*), and glottis (*C*) demonstrate excellent discrimination of mucosa and submucosal tissue, muscle, and lymphoid tissue and salivary glands and subcutaneous tissue.

Specific absorption rate (SAR) refers to the rate at which energy from RF pulses is deposited in the body. SAR increases by a factor of four at 3T compared with 1.5T [2]. RARE sequence, in particular, is affected by the SAR increase because of multiple refocusing pulses. In certain applications it may be necessary to increase the repetition time (TR) or decrease the number of slices to circumvent SAR limitations. SAR also can be mitigated by decreasing the flip angle of refocusing pulses.

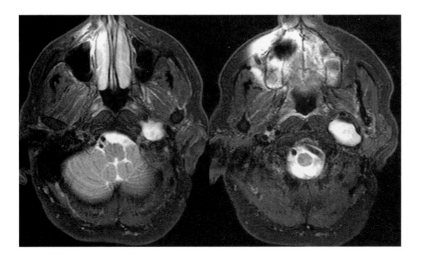

Figure 2 Left jugular foramen schwannoma. Axial T2W images through the skull base show a well-defined and high signal mass in the left jugular foramen with extracranial extension within the carotid sheath. Note the contrast between the nasopharyngeal mucosa and torus tubarius. Asymmetric fat suppression occurred about the right maxilla because of dental filling material.

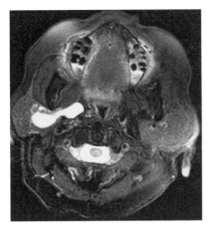

Figure 3 Parotid cyst. Elongated cystic mass in the deep lobe of the parotid with extension into the parapharyngeal space. Exquisite detail of structures with long T2 is provided.

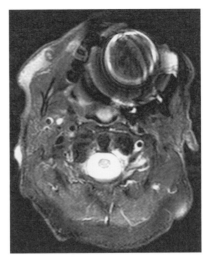

Figure 5 Dental artifacts, which often are nothing more than a nuisance at lower magnetic fields, can prevent evaluation of the oral cavity at 3T.

High spatial resolution images can be obtained by using three-dimensional (3D) spin echo methods, which also minimize some of the disadvantages of two-dimensional sequences (eg, decreased number of slices, SAR concerns); however, the commercial availability of 3D spin echo acquisition methods is limited. Driven equilibrium technique applied to RARE allows scan time reduction; this makes it possible to perform 3D T2W images in acceptable times (Figs. 6–8). This technique provides remarkable signal improvement in tissues with long T1 and T2 (eg, cerebrospinal fluid [CSF]).

High spatial resolution heavily T2W images also can be generated with balanced steady-state gradient-echo imaging (GRE) techniques (aka CISS [constructive interference in the steady state] and FIESTA-C [fast imaging employing steady-state acquisition with phase cycling]). These techniques provide near isotropic voxels and the capability to reconstruct images in any desired plane. Exquisite detail of fluid-containing structures is achieved at the expense of decreased contrast between structures that have intermediate or low T2. Therefore, these sequences are particularly suitable for imaging of the labyrinth, the cochlea, the internal auditory canal (IAC), and the cranial nerves and vessels within the subarachnoid cisterns (Fig. 9).

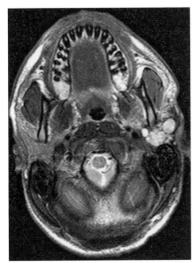

Figure 4 Recurrent mixed adenoma of the parotid. Excellent demonstration of the lobulated nature of the mass.

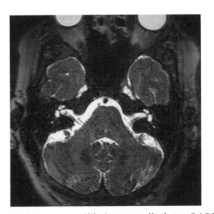

Figure 6 Driven equilibrium applied to RARE sequence allows heavily T2W images of the subarachnoid cisterns (MR-cisternogram). Excellent resolution of the cranial nerves and subarachnoid vessels is achieved. Note a 1-mm vestibular schwannoma associated with the right superior vestibular nerve.

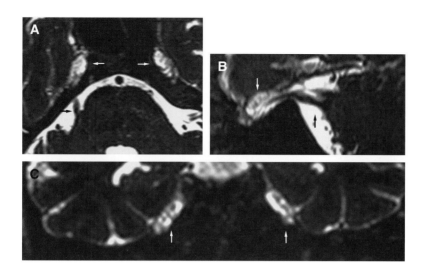

Figure 7 Driven equilibrium applied to RARE sequence allows heavily T2W images of the subarachnoid cisterns (MR-cisternogram). High-quality sagittal oblique (*B*) and coronal (*C*) reconstructions generated from the axially (*A*) obtained data show the cisternal (*black arrows*) and ganglionic parts of the trigeminal nerve. Multiple rootlets (*white arrows*) of the ganglion within the Meckel's cave are demonstrated.

Increasing field strength results in a prolonged T1, which reduces the available signal in short TR sequences. To optimize the tissue contrast on T1W images, modification of TR may be needed that can result in a prolonged acquisition. Many MR imaging practitioners have replaced spin echo T1W images with high spatial resolution 3D spoiled GRE images in brain imaging. It is the authors' opinion that 3D spoiled GRE images are helpful in evaluating the skull base in some clinical scenarios, but spin echo T1W images may prove to be indispensable (Fig. 10). The usefulness/value of T1W 3D spoiled GRE applications in other parts of the head and neck has not been investigated. Alternatively, the use of RARE in T1W imaging is a good compromise between scanning time and contrast. An ETL of 2 or 3 can provide significant time saving with preservation of the contrast that we are accustomed to seeing at the skull base and neck (Fig. 11) [3].

Diffusion-weighted images (DWI) at 3T improved significantly in brain imaging compared with 1.5T because of an increase in SNR. Likewise, perfusion imaging has benefited from increased SNR and increased susceptibility to intravascular contrast material; however we remain challenged in the implementation of these sequences because of the difficulties that are posed by the anatomy of the head and neck. It remains to be proven that gains similar to brain imaging can be realized in head and neck imaging for these applications.

MR spectroscopy is difficult to implement in the head and neck region. The abundance of fat causes fat contamination, which often makes it impossible to interpret the spectra from the lesion of interest. Local field inhomogeneity that is created by bone and air is difficult to correct by shimming. Long scanning time is prohibitive for patients who have airway and swallowing difficulties. One would expect that some of these issues would be addressed with 3T units; however, it is clear that the susceptibility artifacts will continue to be problematic at 3T. Therefore, the authors are not optimistic that high-field imaging will provide any measurable benefit in MR spectroscopy, with the possible exception of large lesions that are distant from the skull base, paranasal sinuses, and mandible.

Coils continue to be just as important as the field strength in high-resolution imaging. An important element of coil design is the number of RF channels that is available for image reconstruction. Eight- and 16-channel coils are commercially available and 64-channel coils are under development. The authors expect to see more multichannel phased-array neck and surface coils becoming commercially available in the near future.

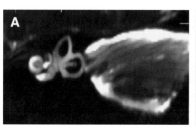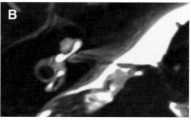

Figure 8 Driven equilibrium applied to RARE sequence allows heavily T2W images of the subarachnoid cisterns. Thick volume reconstruction of the data is used to highlight the membranous labyrinth.

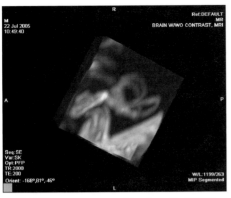

Figure 9 CISS sequence provides heavily T2W images of the subarachnoid cisterns in a similar fashion with the driven equilibrium imaging. Maximum intensity projection (MIP) reconstruction of the data allows 3D visualization of the membranous labyrinth.

Phased-array coils contain multiple coil elements that allow simultaneous data acquisition from large fields of view (FOV) without a decrease in spatial resolution. Parallel imaging techniques (eg, sensitivity encoding [SENSE]) exploit the possibility of using each coil element to reduce the k-space sampling density, and thus, the scanning time. This results in decreased FOV and aliasing. By knowing the spatial sensitivity of each coil element, one can unfold the aliased images and reconstruct the full FOV image. The end result is a significant gain in time and some loss in SNR, which, in some cases, can be alleviated by decreased motion artifacts as a by-product of short scan time or less T2* decay [4,5]. In the author's clinical experience, parallel imaging is problematic in the lower neck because of aliasing that cannot be corrected, whereas the imaging of the skull base is improved by using a head coil.

MR imaging contrast agents are an essential part of head and neck imaging. A new gadolinium-based contrast agent, gadobenate dimeglumine (Gd-BOPTA, Multihance, Bracco, Milan, Italy), recently received U.S. Food and Drug Administration approval. Gd-BOPTA is similar in its physicochemical characteristics to the typical gadolinium-based agents, but it has a much higher relaxivity that provides a higher signal intensity increase. The European experience with Gd-BOPTA showed that it provides a significant advantage [6]. The use of Gd-BOPTA for head and neck imaging at 3T has the potential to improve the visualization of

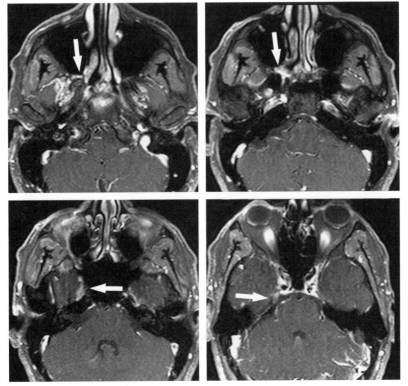

Figure 10 Perineural spread of adenoid cystic cancer of the hard palate. Enhancing tumor (*arrows*) is seen in the pterygopalatine fossa (*top left* and *right*), cavernous sinus, Meckel's cave (*bottom left*), and cisternal portion of the trigeminal nerve (*bottom right*) on conventional spin echo T1W images with fat saturation.

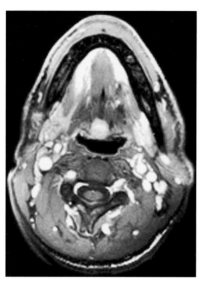

Figure 11 Lingual thyroid. This T1W RARE image was obtained using an ETL of 2.

abnormal enhancement in the cochlea and vestibule. The detection of perineural tumor spread also may benefit from this combination.

Ultrasmall superparamagnetic iron oxide agents, when given intravenously, are taken up by the reticuloendothelial system. They accumulate in the normal lymph nodes, which show a decrease in signal intensity on T2* and T2W MR images because of the susceptibility effect that is created by these particles. Because the susceptibility effects are increased at 3T, these agents may enhance our ability to differentiate normal and abnormal nodes in the head and neck region. The clinical significance of this product remains to be proven.

The clinical application of high field head and neck imaging is an active area of research and published material is scarce.

Lichy and colleagues [7] evaluated the inner ear structures using a 3D CISS sequence and an eight-channel head coil at 1.5T and 3T; they found at least a 30% increase in SNR at 3T. Isotropic voxels provided improved visualization of the vestibule and cochlea. They noted increased pulsation and banding artifacts that did not affect the areas of interest.

Niehues and colleagues [8] compared 3D FIESTA and 3D FIESTA-C sequences using a quadrature head coil and a surface coil at 3T and 1.5T. A combination of a quadrature head coil, FIESTA-C sequence, and imaging at 3T visualized the inner ear and IAC best. Although the surface coil provided high-resolution images of the inner ear at 1.5T and 3T, it failed to demonstrate the IAC and cerebellopontin angle (CPA) at 3T.

Niehues and colleagues [9] demonstrated abnormal enhancement on postcontrast T1W images

at 3T in the vestibules of 20 patients who had Ménière's disease. None of the normal ears in these patients and 20 controls showed a similar enhancement.

Detailed evaluation of the inner ear at 3T is accomplished routinely at the authors' institution. The scala tympani is visualized routinely. This will improve our understanding of conditions, such as Ménière's disease, vertigo, and tinnitus, and provide a better road map for cochlear implantation and endolymphatic sac interventions.

Cramer and colleagues [10] showed improved detection of the intraparotid ductal system at 3T using a balanced GRE and a single-shot RARE sequence. They used a standard head coil for 3T imaging and a phased-array coil for 1.5T imaging.

Orbital imaging also has benefited from the increased SNR and spatial resolution that are associated with the higher field. Using a surface coil, Lemke and colleagues [11] showed improved diagnostic information at 3T, compared with 1.5T, in patients who had uveal melanoma who needed retrobulbar anesthesia to avoid susceptibility artifacts from involuntary eye movements.

Koktzoglou and colleagues [12] compared the SNR efficiency at 1.5T and 3T in carotid artery wall imaging by keeping the spatial resolution and acquisition time constant. They found that 3T imaging provided a 2.2-fold increase in SNR.

DWI has the potential to differentiate malignant and benign tumors in the head and neck region. A significant difference between ADC (apparent diffusion co-efficient) values of malignant tumors and benign conditions of the parotid gland, sinonasal region, and skull base was demonstrated at 1.5T [13]. Sumi and colleagues [14] showed that metastatic lymph nodes in the neck had a higher ADC value than did the normal and lymphomatous nodes. Inflammatory conditions of the parotid gland have higher ADC values than does the normal gland. It is hoped that 3T imaging will provide more insight in this field.

Based on the promise that malignant and benign tissues have different vascular supply, and thus, different enhancement characteristics after contrast administration, investigators evaluated patients who had squamous cell cancer of the neck and nodal metastasis using dynamic contrast-enhanced MR imaging. The slope of the enhancement curve was steeper for the malignant (primary or recurrent) tumors [15]. Fischbein and colleagues [16] reported a surprisingly longer time to peak, lower peak enhancement, lower maximum slope, and slower washout slope in the metastatic nodes compared with the normal nodes. Much work needs to be done in this exciting field. 3T imaging, with its higher capability to demonstrate intravascular susceptibility effects, is expected to improve our understanding of the vascular network of head and neck tumors.

Summary

For the theoretic advantages of 3T units to translate to improved diagnostic quality, careful attention must be paid to optimization of pulse sequences and development of clinically feasible imaging protocols. RARE sequences continue to be the choice for routine clinical imaging of the head and neck; although exquisite T2W images are afforded, T1W imaging is problematic. Short ETL T1W RARE imaging seems to be a good compromise.

References

[1] de Bazelaire CM, Duhamel GD, Rofsky NM, et al. MR imaging relaxation times of abdominal and pelvic tissues measured in vivo at 3.0 T: preliminary results. Radiology 2004;230(3): 652–9.

[2] Lin W, An H, Chen Y, et al. Practical consideration for 3T imaging. Magn Reson Imaging Clin N Am 2003;11:615–39.

[3] DeLano MC, Koon P, Knight TE, et al. 3T imaging of the orbits and internal auditory canals (IAC): fast spin echo sequence optimization. Presented at the American Society of Head and Neck Radiology Annual Meeting. Palm Springs (CA), October 1, 2003.

[4] Pruessmann KP. Parallel imaging at high field strength: synergies and joint potential. Top Magn Reson Imaging 2004;15:237–44.

[5] Pruessmann KP, Weiger M, Scheidegger MB, et al. SENSE: sensitivity encoding for fast MRI. Magn Reson Med 1999;42:952–62.

[6] Proceedings of the MultiHance (gadobenate dimeglumine) user group meeting. December 19–20, 2003. Rome, Italy. Eur Radiol 2004; 14(Suppl 7):O1–88.

[7] Lichy M, Graf H, Damman F, et al. High field MRI of the inner ear. Presented at the Radiological Society of North America's 90th Scientific Assembly and Annual Meeting. Chicago, November 28–December 3, 2004.

[8] Niehues S, Lemke A, Hengst S, et al. Imaging the inner ear and CPA with 1.5 and 3.0 Tesla MRI. Presented at the Radiological Society of North America's 90th Scientific Assembly and Annual Meeting. Chicago, November 28–December 3, 2004.

[9] Niehues S, Lemke A, Hengst S, et al. Imaging the Meniere's disease with 3.0T HR-MRI. Presented at the Radiological Society of North America's 90th Scientific Assembly and Annual Meeting. Chicago, November 28–December 3, 2004.

[10] Cramer M, Habermann J, Graessner J, et al. Comparison of 1.5T and 3T in fast and ultra fast MR sialography. Presented at the Radiological Society of North America's 90th Scientific Assembly and Annual Meeting. Chicago, November 28–December 3, 2004.

[11] Lemke A, Hengst S, Kazi I, et al. First clinical experience with 3.0-T-MRI using a 4-cm surface coil in patients with uveal melanoma. Presented at the Radiological Society of North America's 90th Scientific Assembly and Annual Meeting. Chicago, November 28–December 3, 2004.

[12] Koktzoglou I, Carroll TJ, Walker MT, et al. Multislice carotid wall imaging at 1.5 T and 3.0 T. Presented at the American Society of Neuroradiology's 43rd Annual Meeting. Toronto (Canada), May 21–27, 2005.

[13] AbdelRazek A, El-hawarey G, Shabana Y, et al. Role of diffusion-weighted MR imaging in parotid masses. Presented at the Radiological Society of North America's 90th Scientific Assembly and Annual Meeting. Chicago, November 28–December 3, 2004.

[14] Sumi M, Sakihama N, Sumi T, et al. Discrimination of metastatic cervical lymph nodes with diffusion-weighted MR imaging in patients with head and neck cancer. AJNR Am J Neuroradiol 2003;24:1627–34.

[15] Maroldi R, Farina D, Piazzalunga B. Recurrent head and neck neoplasms: quantitative assessment by means of dynamic MR imaging with analysis of perfusion. Presented at the American Society of Neuroradiology's 43rd Annual Meeting. Toronto (Canada), May 21–27, 2005.

[16] Fischbein NJ, Noworolski SM, Henry RG, et al. Assessment of metastatic cervical adenopathy using dynamic contrast-enhanced MR imaging. AJNR Am J Neuroradiol 2003;24:301–11.

MAGNETIC
RESONANCE
IMAGING CLINICS

Magn Reson Imaging Clin N Am (2006) 97–108

MR Imaging of the Spine at 3T

Marc D. Shapiro MD

Over the past 25 years, MR imaging has evolved into the gold standard for evaluating the bone marrow of the vertebrae and soft tissues within and adjacent to the spine. The soft tissue contrast, direct multiplanar capability, and lack of ionizing radiation with MR imaging contribute to its success as the preferred spine imaging modality. Radiologists and surgeons agree that postmyelographic CT may provide additional diagnostic information under some circumstances (eg, nerve root trauma). Although many clinicians order nuclear medicine bone scans for possible metastatic disease to bone, there is literature to suggest that whole-body T2 STIR (short T1 inversion recovery) MR imaging may be more effective in diagnosing multiple metastases in bone and soft tissues [1].

In recent years, advances in MR imaging technology have led to an increase in scanner field strength, with many institutions upgrading to 3T systems. The first dedicated 3T spine coils were distributed in early 2003. In May 2003, the author's radiology group received the initial first-generation eight-channel, phased array, spine coil. Results on the 3T whole body scanner were discouraging. 3T images of the spine were inferior in quality to those that were obtained on the 1.5T systems.

Other difficulties with first-generation 3T systems included frequent scan interruptions because of radiofrequency (RF) power deposition (specific absorption rate [SAR]) issues, and inadequate

computer processing power that caused 3- to 5-minute delays between pulse sequences on 3T scans when using matrices greater than 256 × 256.

Fortunately, rapid improvements were made in 3T spine imaging technology. In November 2003, the author's facility installed a second-generation 3T MR imaging system with an 8-channel phased array cervical/thoracic/lumbar (CTL) spine coil. The new system had significantly less frequent SAR problems and much improved computer processing power. In the fourth quarter of 2004 a more powerful gradient system and a second-generation 8-channel phased array CTL spine coil were added. These factors further enhanced the quality and speed of the 3T spine imaging. In late 2004, the 3T MR imaging system was upgraded to 16 channels. There are a few 16 and higher channel coils in use in the United States for other anatomic areas, but no 16- or 32-channel spine coils are available. Only theoretic evidence exists to suggest that 16-channel phased array coils will provide significant, if any, improvement, for MR imaging of the spine at 3T.

For more than a year, the author's radiology group has operated four second-generation 3T MR imaging systems; each performs between 25 and 35 scans per day. Thirty-five percent of these procedures are of spines. In stark contrast to the initial experience, the radiologists and referring specialists agree that most spine MR images that are obtained

NeuroSkeletal Imaging Institute of Winter Park, 2111 Glenwood Drive, Winter Park, FL 32792, USA
E-mail address: shapmd@aol.com

doi:10.1016/j.mric.2006.01.005

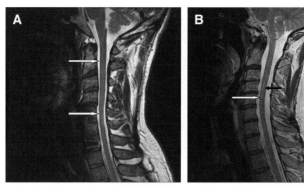

Figure 1 (*A*) Sagittal T2 FSE image, 2-mm slice thickness with 320 × 256 matrices, which are sufficiently high to preclude truncation artifact. Note the visualization of central gray matter or a normal central canal (*white arrows*) in a patient who had a previous anterior fusion. Imaging parameters are adjusted to minimize susceptibility artifact. (*B*) Patient who is asymptomatic and has minimal dilatation of central canal (*black arrow*) posterior to C4 with visualization of normal central canal or central gray matter (*white arrow*) at other levels of cervical spine.

on the author's second-generation 3T systems are superior to those that are obtained on 1.5T systems. The increased signal at 3T provides the primary basis for improved diagnostic quality with clinical efficiency (Fig. 1); however, many challenges accompany the advantages of higher field clinical imaging. Obtaining excellent diagnostic quality with 3T imaging of the spine requires awareness of these challenges and optimization of imaging parameters.

Challenges of 3T spine imaging

The many advantages of higher field clinical imaging are accompanied by novel challenges (compared with imaging at 1.5T) that must be addressed to optimize diagnostic quality. Increased artifacts and RF energy deposition at 3T can be mediated with improved technology of the MR imaging system and surface coils as well as pulse sequence design. In addition, variance in relaxation times between 3T and 1.5T field strengths requires alterations in 1.5T imaging parameters to obtain optimum tissue contrast at 3T.

The resonance frequency, given by the Larmor equation, is proportional to the magnetic field strength. As a result, the increase in field strength from 1.5T to 3T leads to a doubling of the difference in resonance frequency between fat and water protons. This causes misregistration of the data in k-space, and a resulting chemical shift artifact on the image. The chemical shift can be decreased by increasing the receiver bandwidth (RBW); doubling the bandwidth halves the pixel misplacement of fat protons (Fig. 2). Decreasing the field-of-view (FOV) has a similar effect on chemical shift mismapping. Altering either or both of these parameters (increasing RBW or decreasing FOV) also produces a decrease in the signal-to-noise ratio (SNR) that is more pronounced when both parameters are changed; however, it is more than compensated for by the increased signal at 3T.

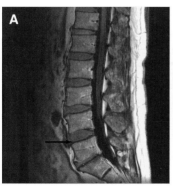
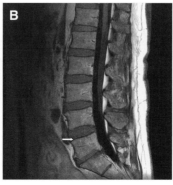

Figure 2 (*A*) Sagittal T1 FLAIR image, 3 mm, matrices 320 × 256, receiver bandwidth 16 kHz. Black arrow points to chemical shift artifact simulating thickened superior endplate of L5. (*B*) Same parameters as (*A*) except bandwidth is increased to 42 kHz. Chemical shift artifact (*white arrow*) is diminished because of the increased bandwidth, which produces less pixel misregistration.

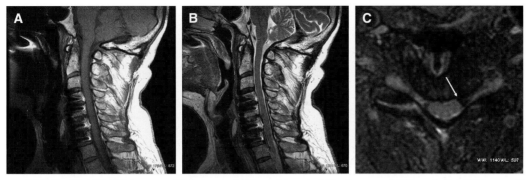

Figure 3 (*A*) Sagittal T1 FSE image with increased ETL and bandwidth decreased ETL and slice thickness. Note orientation of frequency encoding parallel to the longest axis of the hardware. More then adequate visualization of cervical spinal cord is possible when the five imaging parameters are adjusted properly. (*B*) Sagittal T2 FSE image with increased ETL and bandwidth, and decreased TE and slice thickness. Again, frequency encoding is parallel to longest axis of the metal hardware. (*C*) Axial T2 FSE image with fat saturation. Susceptibility artifact is mitigated, which permits visualization of entire cord and the right nerve root; however, artifact does encroach on the proximal portion (*arrow*) of the left nerve root.

Static field inhomogeneity and susceptibility

Susceptibility to magnetic field heterogeneity increases with increasing field strength. In addition, at 3T there is shortening of T2 and T2*, which produces greater signal dropout and geometric distortion. Susceptibility must be mitigated for optimized image quality at 3T in patients with spine hardware; there are many available techniques for combating susceptibility challenges. Increasing the RBW and maximizing the echo train length (ETL), decreasing the slice thickness and echo time (TE) and orienting the frequency-encoding direction parallel to the long axis of any metal will diminish susceptibility artifact (Fig. 3) [2]. When selecting a 3T system, users who will be imaging postoperative spines with any frequency should take into consideration a system's ability to change these imaging parameters readily on multiple sequences. Also of significance, fast spin echo (FSE) or turbo spin echo sequences display less susceptibility than do conventional spin echo (CSE) sequences. Gradient echo (GRE) sequences exacerbate susceptibility artifact and should be avoided, if possible, when imaging patients with

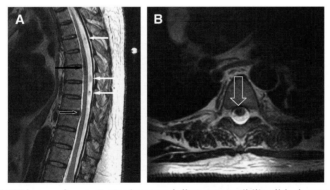

Figure 4 (*A*) Sagittal T2 FSE image demonstrates intramedullary susceptibility (*black arrow*) that probably is due to hemosiderin associated with old hemorrhage in a patient who had normal cord signal on 1.5T MR image 6 months earlier. Susceptibility is increased significantly at 3T. There are flow artifacts (*white arrows*) within the posterior subarachnoid space. Flow and pulsation artifacts also are exacerbated at 3T. Note small disc protrusion (*outlined black arrow*) as well. (*B*) Axial T2 FSE image with fat saturation again demonstrates two foci of susceptibility (*arrow*) within the thoracic cord that probably are related to hemosiderin. If one used a GRE axial pulse sequence the area of susceptibility would increase (bloom) in size. FSE (turbo spin echo) sequences with a long ETL and short TE help to decrease susceptibility.

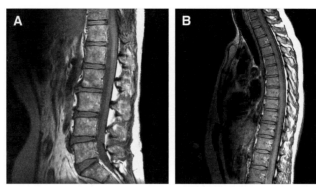

Figure 5 (A) Sagittal T1 FSE image of the lumbar spine. At 3T, tissues and fluids (not containing methemoglobin or high protein content which would shorten T1 relaxivity) have prolonged T1 relaxation times. If spin echo (FSE and CSE) sequences are used for T1-weighted images, the normal interfaces between cord, conus, and cauda equina and CSF that are seen at 1.5T and lower field strengths are blurred secondary to increased signal of fluid at 3T. If this increased signal of the CSF were present at lower field strength it would suggest pathology. (B) 3T sagittal T1 FSE image of thoracic spine. The effect of prolonged T1 relaxation times again demonstrates blurring of the margins (the anterior border suffers more in this image) between spinal cord and CSF. The proximal cauda equina is poorly differentiated from CSF.

spine hardware at 3T. The author failed to produce diagnostic-quality MR images in only 3 out of more than 700 postoperative spine patients who were imaged on his 3T systems. All three had the same metal cage. Subsequently, these patients were imaged on a 0.7T system, which also failed to provide a diagnostic-quality examination secondary to excessive magnetic susceptibility artifacts. The increased susceptibility at 3T can be helpful in some circumstances, and results in improved detection of hemosiderin or calcification (Fig. 4).

Flow artifacts

Flow and pulsation artifacts also increase with increasing field strength and are exacerbated significantly at 3T. This may obscure pathology (including abnormal enhancement) on T1-weighted spin echo pulse sequences, particularly with T1-FSE sequences, but also with CSE sequences. All manufacturers' 3T systems have only unidirectional flow compensation which, when used, necessitates an increase in minimum TE.

Table 1:   **Noncontrast lumbar spine scans**

	Series 1	Series 2	Series 3	Series 4	Series 5	Series 6
Series description	T1 FLAIR	Sag T2 FSE	Axial T2 FSE	Axial T1 FSE	Post T1 FLAIR	Post Axial T1 FSE
Scan plane	Sag	Sag	Oblique	Oblique	Sag	Oblique
TE (ms)	17	85	85	min	17	min
TR (ms)	2675	3325	3800	80	2675	80
TI	2000				2000	
Echo train length	7	18	18	3	7	3
Receive bandwidth (kHz)		32	32	32		32
FOV (mm)		26	18	18		18
Scan thickness (mm)	3	3	3	3	3	3
Interscan spacing (mm)	1	1	1	1	1	1
Frequency (matrix)	320	416	256	256	320	256
Phase (matrix)	256	289	224	224	256	224
NEX	2	3	2	2	2	2
Contrast					Yes	Yes
Time	3:55	2:46	3:33	6:05	3:55	6:05

Abbreviations: NEX, number of excitations; Sag, sagittal.

Table 2: **Noncontrast cervical spine scans**

	Series 1	Series 2	Series 3
Series description	T1 FLAIR	Sag T2 FSE	Axial T2 FSE FS
Scan plane	Sag	Sag	Oblique
TE/TE2 (ms)	17	85	85
TR (ms)	2675	3000	4000
TI/TI 2	2000		
Echo train length	7	16	18
Receive bandwidth (kHz)	32	32	32
SATS			Fat classic
FOV (mm)		21	16
Scan thickness (mm)	3	3	3
Interscan spacing (mm)	1	0.3	0.3
Frequency (matrix)	320	256	256
Phase (matrix)	256	256	256
NEX	2	3	3
Time	3:55	2:51	5:38

Abbreviations: NEX, number of excitations; Sag, sagittal.

The quality of spine MR imaging at any field strength is improved by placing saturation bands above pulsatile vessels and between these vessels and the important anatomic structures; this is even more effective with 3T systems. Additionally, avoiding the use of the anteroposterior (AP) direction for phase encoding for spine MR imaging helps to prevent these artifacts from obscuring the spinal cord and proximal nerve roots.

Specific absorption rate management

The increase in the resonance frequency at 3T causes increased energy deposition in body tissues, which is measured and reported as SAR. This is a particular problem on large FOV scans, such as an MR metastatic survey of the entire spine (FOV, 45–50 cm), and with FSE or turbo spin echo sequences where the problem is exacerbated by using shorter repetition times (TRs) and more RF pulses. Parallel imaging (PI) techniques can reduce SAR effectively (see later discussion). GRE sequences are best for minimizing SAR. CSE sequences are less SAR intensive than are FSE sequences [2]. Other SAR-friendly manipulations include reducing the ETL and increasing the TR for any FSE (turbo spin echo) sequence.

T1-weighted spine imaging

Perhaps the major challenge of spine imaging at 3T is related to the increased T1 relaxation times. The

Table 3: **Noncontrast thoracic spine scans**

	Series 1	Series 2	Series 3
Series description	T1 FLAIR	Sag T2 FSE	Axial T2 FSE
Scan plane	Sag	Sag	Oblique
TE/TE2 (ms)	17	85	85
TR (ms)	2500	2750	3350
TI/TI 2	2000		
Echo train length	7	18	18
Receive bandwidth (kHz)	32	32	32
FOV (mm)		32	20
Scan thickness (mm)	3	3	3
Interscan spacing (mm)	1	1	1
Frequency (matrix)	320	416	256
Phase (matrix)	256	288	224
NEX	2	3	3
Time	3:55	2:18	4:35

Abbreviations: NEX, number of excitations; Sag, sagittal.

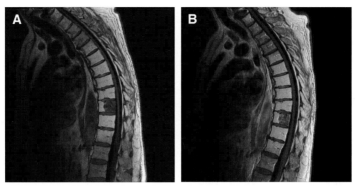

Figure 6 (*A*) 3T sagittal T1 FLAIR image of thoracic spine in a patient who has prostate cancer represents a good example of differentiating between almost normal (except that the T1 signal intensity is too high relative to excess yellow marrow) and obviously abnormal bone marrow signal intensity. The fatty infiltration of bone marrow can be related to aging or radiation changes. Note flow artifacts that are exacerbated at 3T within the posterior subarachnoid space. (*B*) 3T sagittal T1 FLAIR image after intravenous gadolinium (half standard dose at 0.05 mmol/kg) demonstrates some enhancement within this biopsy-proven solitary metastasis. A similar enhancement pattern can be seen in hemangiomas.

longer T1 times cause the signal intensity of cerebrospinal fluid (CSF) to change from dark at low field strength to gray at 3T. If CSF is gray for 3T spine imaging, the interpreter loses normal T1 interfaces between cord, conus, cauda equina, and CSF (Fig. 5). The decreased fluid–tissue contrast makes detection of subarachnoid involvement with infectious, inflammatory, or neoplastic diseases formidable if noncontrast T1 FSE or CSE sequences alone are used at 3T. With intravenous contrast, detection of small tumors becomes possible.

The use of GRE pulse sequences can diminish problems that are associated with lengthened T1 relaxation times. The best CSF–soft tissue contrast for T1-weighted spine imaging at 3T is achieved with T1 FLAIR (fluid-attenuated inversion recovery)

pulse sequences. This sequence was tried previously at 1.5T with early promising results, but it never achieved widespread use. The author and colleagues [3] prospectively compared noncontrast spine scans with T1 FLAIR and T1 FSE in the sagittal plane of 110 patients (50 lumbar, 50 cervical, and 10 thoracic; Tables 1–3). The parameters evaluated included cord, conus, and cauda equina interfaces with CSF, vertebral body, and disc–CSF interfaces; differentiation between normal and abnormal bone marrow (Figs. 6 and 7); magnetic susceptibility artifact size from spine hardware; detection of abnormal intramedullary signal; and the ability and quality of chemical fat saturation. The results showed that T1 FLAIR is better than T1 FSE in delineating all normal tissues interfaces between soft

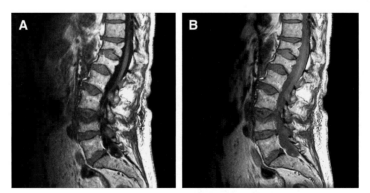

Figure 7 (*A*) 3T sagittal T1 FLAIR image of lumbar spine demonstrates again how well this pulse sequence delineates abnormal bone marrow signal, this time in an acute nonneoplastic vertebral body compression fracture. There also are old nonneoplastic compression fractures. (*B*) Sagittal T1 FSE demonstrates the same findings as in (*A*), but the conus medullaris and cauda equina are not delineated well secondary to the prolonged T1 relaxation time and increased (gray) signal of the CSF on FSE and CSE pulse sequences.

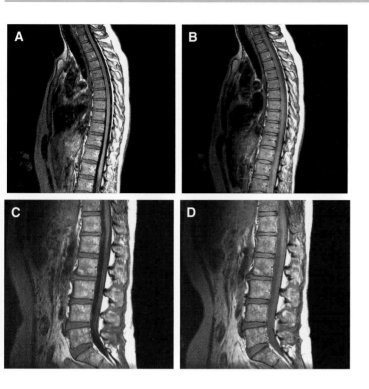

Figure 8 (*A*) Sagittal T1 FLAIR image of thoracic spine illustrates how well the interfaces between the spinal cord and CSF are delineated on T1 FLAIR sequences. (*B*) 3T sagittal T1 FSE image of the thoracic spine does not delineate CSF–cord interfaces nearly as well as in (*A*) because of increased CSF signal on spin echo sequences. (*C*) 3T sagittal T1 FLAIR image of the lumbar spine demonstrates excellent delineation of the distal cauda equina and conus are with darker CSF produced by this sequence. (*D*) 3T sagittal T1 FSE image for comparison with T1 FLAIR image (*C*). The distal cauda equina is blurred secondary to the gray signal of CSF with T1 spin echo sequences at 3T.

tissue–CSF–bone or disc–CSF as well as abnormal–normal tissue interfaces (Fig. 8). T1 FLAIR also is superior for mitigating susceptibility artifact because of its longer ETL (7 versus 2).

Contrast enhancement

The ability to demonstrate contrast enhancement adequately is of major significance for any T1-weighted pulse sequence. During the past 2 years, the author and colleagues [4,5] conducted two separate, prospective, 100-patient studies on 3T systems. They evaluated for number and conspicuity of contrast-enhancing lesions in the brain by comparing T1 FSE with three-dimensional (3D) FSPGR (fast spoiled gradient-recalled acquisition into steady state) and then evaluated the same parameters by comparing T1 CSE with T1 FLAIR. The readers could not be double blinded on either study because of the marked disparity in gray–white matter contrast between the pulse sequences. Most lesions were well delineated and equally conspicuous on all sequences; however, some varied in appearance (ring versus solid) and conspicuity on the pulse sequences. A small number of clinically significant lesions, including a small metastasis, several active demyelinating plaques, and a few occult cerebral vascular malformations (OCVMs), were identified on FSE or CSE that were missed with T1 FLAIR or T1 FSPGR (Figs. 9 and 10).

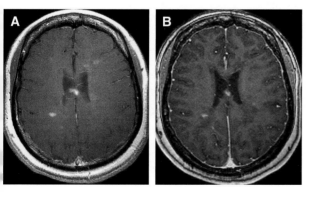

Figure 9 (*A*) 3T axial T1 FSE image after contrast demonstrates several active demyelinating plaques that are not visualized on T1 FSPGR image (*B*). (*B*) 3T axial T1 FSPGR image with fewer and some less conspicuous enhancing, active multiple sclerosis plaques. Spin echo (CSE and FSE) at 3T improves the conspicuity of enhancement compared with background, because of the suppression effect of prolonged T1 relaxation time of tissue at this field strength.

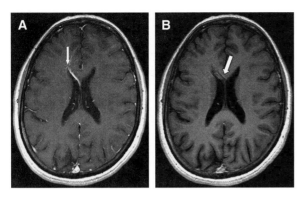

Figure 10 (*A*) 3T axial T1 postcontrast CSE image delineates the venous angioma (DVA) of left frontal lobe (*arrow*). Again, the background suppression related to prolonged T1 relaxation times is most pronounced on T1 spin echo sequences. (*B*) 3T postgadolinium axial T1 FLAIR sequence shows poor enhancement of same DVA (*arrow*) as in (*A*). This may be misinterpreted as normal increased flow artifact at 3T. Note improved gray–white matter delineation of T1 FLAIR sequence when compared with T1 CSE in (*A*).

In contradistinction to the above, some OCVMs were seen on FSPGR and were missed on T1 FSE. These findings prompted the investigators to obtain at least one FSE (usually) or CSE sequence in one plane on all contrast-enhanced MR imaging examinations of the brain and spine at 3T (Fig. 11). In the authors' experience on all field strength scanners, the conspicuity of enhancement is at least as dependent on the time interval between injection and imaging. Improved conspicuity of abnormal enhancing tissue is seen almost always on the more delayed pulse sequence (Fig. 12). The author and colleagues just completed a prospective postcontrast comparison between T1 FSE and T1 FLAIR pulse sequences for the number and conspicuity of enhancing abnormalities in 110 patients who were imaged at 3T. In 55 patients spines were imaged with sagittal T1 FSE obtained before sagittal T1 FLAIR, whereas 55 patients had the sagittal T1 FLAIR performed as the initial postcontrast

sequence. In 70% of the spines both sagittal sequences were imaged using fat saturation. All axial T1-weighed images were performed with a T1 FSE sequence.

The results demonstrated 56 abnormalities that showed pathologic enhancement. No enhancing pathology was delineated on only one of the two T1 pulse sequences. Variation in the conspicuity of enhancement was solely dependent on, and improved with, the sequence obtained with a longer interval between injection and imaging (Fig. 13) [3].

Advantages of 3T spine imaging

The theoretic SNR of 3T imaging is twice that of 1.5T imaging. As a result, the increased signal can be traded for other qualities to optimize image quality and efficiency. Thinner anatomic slices at 3T maintain the same or greater SNR as on the same

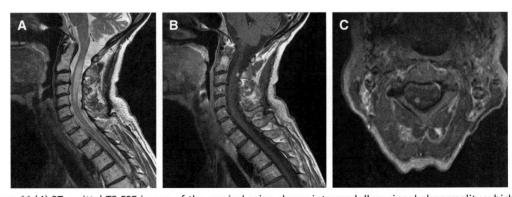

Figure 11 (*A*) 3T sagittal T2 FSE image of the cervical spine shows intramedullary signal abnormality which has a nodule of enhancement in the right posterior aspect of the cord on T1 FLAIR sagittal (*B*) and T1 FSE axial (*C*) images. Biopsy-proven hemangioblastoma. (*B*) 3T sagittal T1 FLAIR image after contrast with extensive pulsation artifacts makes this look more like a T1 FSE image. (*C*) 3T axial T1 FSE image after contrast shows the nodule of enhancement seen in (*B*). Note extensive pulsation artifacts that are increased at 3T, especially on FSE sequences.

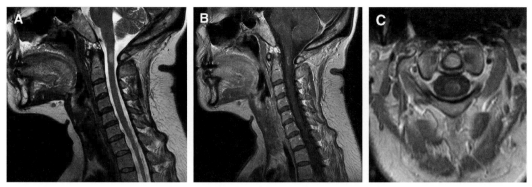

Figure 12 (*A*) 3T sagittal T2 FSE image in patient who has multiple sclerosis (MS) demonstrates a typical, almost flame-shaped intramedullary signal abnormality in the posterior half of spinal cord at C2 level. This is a common location for demyelinating plaques in MS to involve the cord. 3T sagittal (*B*) and axial (*C*) T1 FSE images after gadolinium contrast demonstrate rim enhancement of T2 hyperintensity at C2, which is indicative of an active demyelinating plaque. The rim of enhancement may fill with contrast on delayed postgadolinium images. The conspicuity of enhancement increases at 3T because of prolonged T1 relaxation of tissue.

scan that is obtained on a 1.5T system. Specifically, slice thickness at 3T can be halved by using the same matrices as at 1.5T. This can be particularly helpful with thin-section 3D pulse sequences of the cervical spine predominantly for the axial plane (Fig. 14). The extra signal also can be used to double matrix sizes, and thereby, increase spatial resolution, while maintaining the same slice thickness that is used for 1.5T (Fig. 15). Another option at 3T is to maintain the same spatial resolution and SNR for imaging at 1.5T, and reduce scan times by a factor of four compared with those used at 1.5T.

PI techniques, which reduce the number of phase-encoding lines in k space by substituting spatial encoding information that is afforded by the phased array coils sensitivity profiles, offer a synergistic improvement when combined with 3T technology [6]. By reducing the number of phase-encoding steps, PI techniques reduce scan time and permit the imager to decrease the ETL, which in turn, reduces SAR. PI techniques diminish SAR because of the reduced number of transmitted RF pulses to the patient's body, which is particularly important at higher field strength. A loss in overall SNR accompanies PI techniques; the amount of decrease in SNR depends on which acceleration factor (2, 3, 4, or 6) is used to obtain the scan. The increased SNR at 3T makes the decrease in SNR (40% and 50% for acceleration factors of 2 and 3)

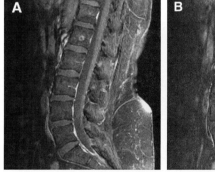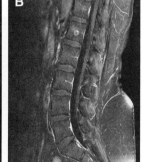

Figure 13 3T postcontrast, fat-suppressed sagittal T1 FSE (*A*) and T1 FLAIR (*B*) images demonstrate excellent chemically selected fat saturation, which is more robust at 3T because of the greater separation of resonance peaks in fat and water. Enhancement within a high-intensity zone seen on T2-weighted images in the posterior aspect of the L3–4 intervertebral disc. Most frequently, this represents a tear of the annular fibers that usually is not an acute finding. Note the rounded area of enhancement in the L1 vertebral body, which is related to contrast in the basivertebral plexus or in a small hemangioma. The enhancement on the cord's posterior surface and in the cauda equina is due to normal vessels that are seen commonly on 3T images with contrast.

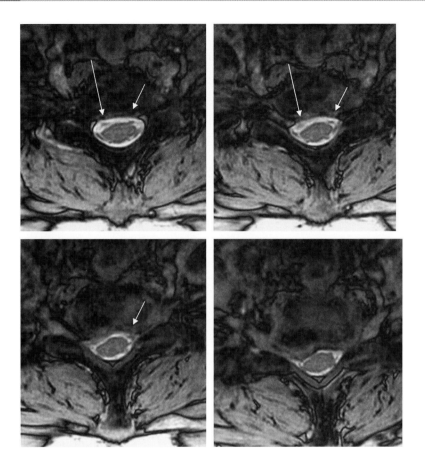

Figure 14 3T COSMIC 3D axial GRE images. The development of new pulse sequences, such as COSMIC with high spatial resolution and excellent SNR, depict CSF–spinal cord interfaces and differentiate discs (higher in signal intensity from osteophyte). Thinner slices also help to provide more detail of the foramina. Note that the right anterior C8 root is compressed (*arrows*). (Courtesy of Mark DeLano, MD, Michigan State University, East Lansing, MI.)

associated with PI tolerable. Another benefit to imaging at 3T is the increased conspicuity of paramagnetic contrast agents on T1-weighted images (Fig. 16) [7]. T1 relaxation times of tissues and fluids are prolonged at 3T, which results in suppression of signal from noncontrast-enhanced tissue. The effect is analogous to magnetization transfer pulses that are used for background suppression. The increased conspicuity of contrast agents at 3T has permitted the use of half

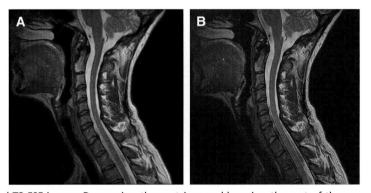

Figure 15 3T sagittal T2 FSE image. Decreasing the matrices and keeping the rest of the parameters constant at a given field strength result in higher SNR with decreased spatial resolution. (*A*) 320 × 256. (*B*) Lower SNR with improved spatial resolution after increasing the matrix to 512 × 384 and maintaining other parameters, including field strength. If the field strength is doubled (1.5T to 3T) and slice thickness remains constant, the matrices can be doubled without decreasing SNR.

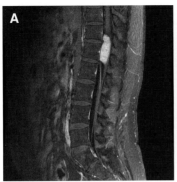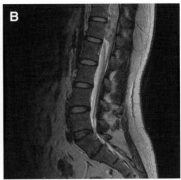

Figure 16 3T sagittal postcontrast T1 FLAIR (*A*) and sagittal T2 FSE (*B*) images in a patient who had a myxopapillary ependymoma in this tumor's most common location within the proximal cauda equina. There is robust enhancement with half the standard dose (sd = 0.1 mmol/kg) after contrast, which is more pronounced at 3T than at 1.5T. Note enhancement in the nerve root which is displaced anteriorly by the tumor.

(0.05 mmol/kg) of the standard dose of contrast (1 mmol/kg) [8].

The increased chemical shift at 3T allows for improved chemically selective fat saturation pulses (Fig. 17), which can be used to mediate some of the artifacts and contrast issues that are associated with high-field imaging. A limited number of institutions perform spinal cord diffusion imaging, diffusion tensor imaging, and spectroscopy at 3T. These techniques show promise and likely will proliferate in the next few years. In addition, increased coil density, with 16- and 32-channel phased array spine coils, probably will come to fruition, which will improve spine imaging at 3T.

Summary

There are many advantages and challenges associated with 3T imaging of the spine. The increase in SNR allows for optimization of diagnostic quality

and improved clinical efficiency. PI techniques merge well with high-field technology, which minimizes many of the challenges that are associated with 3T systems. The increase in chemical shift, pulsatile flow, and susceptibility artifact can be mediated with manipulation of imaging parameters. One major challenge that plagued 3T imaging of the spine was the decrease in fluid contrast that was associated with the lengthened T1 relaxation times. This has been resolved essentially for noncontrast spine imaging by using T1 FLAIR, which delineates soft tissue, CSF, disc, and bone interfaces exquisitely well. The optimal postcontrast T1 sequence may not exist yet. Clinical experience dictates that with a combination of T1 FLAIR with or without fat saturation (in one plane) and T1 FSE (in the other plane) no significant enhancing pathology will be missed. Despite the challenges, 3T imaging of the spine provides many improvements over 1.5T systems. These advances can be

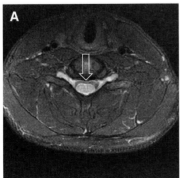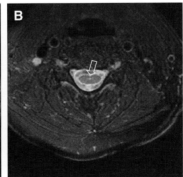

Figure 17 (*A*) 3T two-dimensional axial T2 FSE image with fat suppression demonstrates that the normal-sized central canal (*arrow*) is barely perceptible. Note the excellent delineation of nerve roots within the foramina. Chemically selective fat saturation is uniform and reliable at 3T. (*B*) 3T 3D MERGE (multiple echo recombination of gradient echoes) shows minimally dilated central canal (*arrow*), which is essentially normal (≤2 mm) in an asymptomatic patient.

maximized by use of still evolving technologies and pulse sequence designs.

References

[1] Walker R, Kessar P, Blanchard R, et al. Turbo STIR magnetic resonance imaging as a whole-body screening tool for metastases in patients with breast carcinoma: preliminary clinical experience. J Magn Reson Imaging 2000;11(4):343–50.

[2] Lin W, An H, Chen Y, et al. Practical consideration for 3T imaging. Magn Reson Imaging Clin N Am 2003;11(4):615–39.

[3] Shapiro MD, Hartker R, Williams D. Post contrast imaging of the spine at 3T: T1 FLAIR vs. T1 FSE. Presented at the 44th ASNR Annual Meeting. San Diego.

[4] Shapiro MD, Hartker R, Williams D, et al. Post contrast imaging of the brain at 3T: T1 FLAIR vs. T1 CSE: which pulse sequence should we use? Presented at the 44th ASNR Annual Meeting. San Diego.

[5] Shapiro MD, Ramnath RR, Williams D. The conspicuity of paramagnetic contrast enhancement of the brain at 3Tesla: 3D FSPGR vs 2D Ti FSE. Presented at the 90th Scientific Assembly of the Radiologic Society of North America. Chicago.

[6] Pruessmann KP. Parallel imaging at high field strength: synergies and joint potential. Top Magn Reson Imaging 2004;15(4):237–44.

[7] Shapiro MD, Ramnath RR, Williams D. T1 FLAIR vs. T1 FSE: the optimal T1 pulse sequence for clinical spine imaging at 3T. Presented at the 43rd ASNR Annual Meeting. Toronto.

[8] Krautmacher C, Willinek WA, Tschampa HJ, et al. Brain tumors: full- and half-dose contrast-enhanced MR imaging at 3.0 T compared with 1.5 T–initial experience. Radiology 2005; 237(3):1014–9.

Magn Reson Imaging Clin N Am (2006) 109–121

ELSEVIER
SAUNDERS

Extracranial Carotid MR Imaging at 3T

J. Kevin DeMarco MD[a],*, John Huston III MD[b],
Andrew K. Nash MS[c]

- Review of current literature about 1.5T carotid contrast-enhanced MR angiography
- Implications for extracranial carotid MR angiography at 3T
- 3T carotid contrast-enhanced MR angiography and plaque imaging using dedicated surface coils
- Initial clinical experience with 500- to 600-μm carotid contrast-enhanced MR angiography at 3T
- Initial clinical experience with carotid plaque imaging in vivo at 3T
- Initial clinical experience with large field-of-view carotid contrast-enhanced MR angiography at 3T
- Summary
- References

There is clear evidence from multiple carotid trials, including a recent pooled data analysis, that surgical intervention with carotid endarterectomy has significant benefits compared with medical therapy in symptomatic patients who have severe carotid stenosis [1–3]. Intra-arterial digital subtraction angiography (DSA) has been the gold standard for measuring the carotid stenosis in these trials. The improved efficacy of noninvasive imaging techniques and the attendant risk of stoke during the DSA led many practices to adopt noninvasive modalities, such as Doppler ultrasound (US), MR angiography, or CT angiography (CTA), to replace this invasive study. Carotid stenosis evaluation has been a major driving force in developing MR angiography.

Despite the availability of high-quality US, CTA, and MR angiography, no consensus exists regarding the optimal noninvasive imaging strategy for the preoperative evaluation of carotid stenosis. This is particularly true for MR angiography. In the 1990s, time-of-flight (TOF) MR angiography was reported to have good sensitivity and specificity in detecting internal carotid artery stenosis of more than 70% using North American Symptomatic Carotid Endarterectomy Trial Criteria (NASCET) criteria identified on DSA [4–6]. Contrast-enhanced (CE) MR angiography offered the opportunity to cover more of the carotid artery distribution in a fraction of the time that TOF MR angiography required. With the advent of elliptic-centric phase reordering and effective timing of the gadolinium contrast bolus, first-pass CE MR angiography moved from research into routine clinical practice. Despite abundant literature, the optimal imaging strategy for carotid MR angiography remains controversial. Some investigators insist that with today's techniques, TOF MR angiography remains the most accurate technique [7]. For those who prefer CE MR angiography, three competing

[a] Department of Radiology, Michigan State University, 184 Radiology Building, East Lansing, MI 48824, USA
[b] MR Research Lab, Mayo Clinic, Rochester, MN, USA
[c] College of Human Medicine, Michigan State University, East Lansing, MI, USA
*Corresponding author.
E-mail address: jkd@rad.msu.edu (J.K. DeMarco).

doi:10.1016/j.mric.2005.12.003

techniques evolved. One approach uses multiple time points during the gadolinium bolus arrival with multiple rapid three-dimensional (3D) acquisitions with low spatial resolution. To achieve a higher spatial resolution and improved temporal resolution, 3D acquisitions reconstructed with a novel oversampling of the center of k-space are possible. This technique is termed "time-resolved intravascular contrast kinetics." As experience with gadolinium bolus arrival timing improved, many investigators abandoned the time-resolved approach to carotid CE MR angiography in favor of a higher spatial resolution technique. The use of elliptic-centric phase reordering in combination with a bolus arrival scan or fluoroscopic triggering allowed carotid CE MR angiography with 45- to 60-second scan duration with good intra-arterial contrast and little venous contamination. The spatial resolution of these longer acquisitions was superior to the time-resolved carotid CE MR angiography. To decrease motion artifact, the elliptic-centric phase reordering sequence can be shortened by up to 50% with the tradeoff of lower spatial resolution. There also is less stress placed on the exact gadolinium bolus arrival timing by providing a shorter scan with less sensitivity to venous contamination. An extensive study of the tradeoffs between shorter scan time and less spatial resolution compared with longer scan time and higher spatial resolution for carotid elliptic-centric phase reordered CE MR angiography does not exist. This limitation may help to explain the current controversy surrounding the best carotid MR angiography technique.

Review of current literature about 1.5T carotid contrast-enhanced MR angiography

The current controversy about carotid CE MR angiography may be illustrated best by reviewing two recent publications in 2005. Willinek and colleagues [8] reported on a prospective comparison of 50 consecutive patients who underwent CE MR angiography and DSA for the detection of steno-occlusive disease of the supra-aortic arteries. They listed CE MR angiography as having a sensitivity of 100% (73/73) and a specificity of 99.3% (760/765) in detecting 70% to 99% diameter stenosis that was identified on DSA. Although some investigators might argue that this reported specificity was elevated by the inclusion of other arteries in addition to the internal carotid artery, the reported accuracy—when limited to the internal carotid artery stenosis—remained high. The investigators used a 58-second scan with submillimeter in-plane resolution and 1-mm through-plane resolution. Specifically, the coronally acquired field of view (FOV) was 350 mm with a matrix of 432 × 432. Sixty partitions, each 1-mm thick, covered the 60-mm thick

slab in the anteroposterior (AP) direction, which resulted in a prescribed matrix size of 0.81 × 0.81 × 1.0 mm. A percentage decrease in the actual acquired-phase encoding steps exactly matched the decrease in FOV in the phase direction. This allowed the prescribed voxel resolution to remain as stated while decreasing the acquisition time to 58 seconds. A double dose of an extracellular gadolinium contrast agent was used along with a commercially available phased-array coil that covered the upper chest, neck, and head in a modern 1.5T MR scan with high performance gradients, including a 30 mT/m gradient amplitude.

Different conclusions regarding the efficacy of CE MR angiography were reported in an article that was published in 2005 by Fellner and colleagues [9]. They used an unenhanced TOF MR angiogram, a first-pass CE MR angiogram with fluoroscopic triggering, and a time-resolved CE MR angiogram. The time-resolved sequence consisted of a second contrast bolus and four data sets which each lasted for 10 seconds and resulted in less spatial resolution compared with the first-pass CE MR angiogram. Their results indicated a slightly higher correlation between DSA and first-pass CE MR angiogram compared with the time-resolved technique. Although both techniques were 100% sensitive, the specificity of TOF MR angiography was superior to first-pass CE MR angiography in depicting severe carotid stenosis as seen on DSA (96.7% versus 80.6%). The investigators recommended TOF MR angiography and first-pass CE MR angiography in the preoperative evaluation of carotid stenosis. Review of first-pass CE MR angiography protocol revealed some interesting differences compared with the data of Willinek and colleagues [8]. Most striking was the much shorter scan time of 31 seconds. Although there is the potential for less motion artifact compared with the longer protocol that was used by Willinek and colleagues, the spatial resolution also is decreased. A FOV of 187.5 × 300 mm was used for first-pass CE MR angiogram with a matrix of 160 × 512, which results in a prescribed pixel size of 0.6 × 1.2 mm. The investigators listed a measured slice thickness of 1.3 mm. The actual thickness of the coronal slab acquisition and number of acquired phase steps in the z direction were not listed. The voxel size that was used by Fellner and colleagues (0.6 × 1.2 × 1.3 mm) is more anisotropic compared with the one that was used by Willinek and colleagues (0.81 × 0.81 × 1.0 mm). The resulting voxel volume—as measured before any interpolation—that was used by Fellner and colleagues (0.94 mm^3) was larger than that used by Willinek and colleagues (0.66 mm^3). In a review of 20 recent publications [8–27] that compared first-pass CE MR angiography with DSA, 6 studies reported high sensitivity, but low specificity of CE MR angiography in detecting severe stenosis as seen on DSA. All six of the studies used scan times of less than 45 seconds for the CE MR angiography, and none used submillimeter to millimeter in-plane resolution combined with 1.0- to 1.2-mm partition thickness.

Based upon the published data, it is reasonable to conclude that longer (50–60 seconds) scan times with first-pass CE MR angiography result in more accurate examinations that yield better correlation with DSA than do shorter (<45 seconds) scans that do not include parallel imaging techniques. Although examination times of 30 seconds or less may allow a breath-hold acquisition, the higher spatial resolution of 50- to 60-second scans seems to be more important in the accurate identification of carotid stenosis at the bifurcation. This is in keeping with the initial simulations of first-pass elliptic-centric phase reordered CE MR angiography that predicted the best performance with high resolution, while maintaining a minimum-phase FOV in the y and z directions [28]. A three-way prospective study of a longer (50–60 seconds) first-pass CE MR angiogram, a 30-second CE MR angiogram, and a noncontrast TOF MR angiogram compared with the "gold standard" rotational DSA in the preoperative evaluation of carotid stenosis would determine which technique is superior, if the study included a sufficiently large number of patients. In the absence of such a study, the above analysis suggests that higher spatial resolution first-pass CE MR angiography, perhaps combined with TOF MR angiography, is the best technique to depict carotid stenosis at the carotid bifurcation.

This analysis does not take into account the appearance of the take-off of the great vessels from the arch that should be depicted better during a breath-hold acquisition. If there is too much motion artifact on the 50- to 60-second CE MR angiogram to visualize the great vessels, a second, smaller gadolinium bolus injection during a breath-hold CE MR angiogram may be helpful. Experience has shown that a second gadolinium injection has an acceptable minimal venous contamination from the first injection on repeat CE MR angiograms. In the authors' experience with more than 3000 CE MR angiograms, the take-off of the great vessels can be visualized adequately on a 50- to 60-second CE MR angiogram by reviewing the source coronal images as well as multiplanar reformations in the left anterior oblique (LAO) projection.

Implications for extracranial carotid MR angiography at 3T

Missing from this initial discussion of extracranial carotid CE MR angiography at 1.5T are the important factors of signal-to-noise ratio (SNR) and contrast-to-noise ratio (CNR). It is imperative that adequate SNR/CNR be obtained to generate good image quality (IQ), with the recommended submillimeter to millimeter in-plane resolution and 1.0- to 1.2-mm through-plane resolution CE MR angiography. In general, CE MR angiography is a high SNR/CNR technique. Pushing spatial resolution to these recommended levels requires a good deal of attention to technique, modern equipment, and adequate timing of a large bolus of gadolinium contrast. All major MR manufacturers offer eight-channel or higher neurovascular coils for 1.5T MR scanners. In addition, most investigators now use a double dose of extracellular gadolinium contrast agents or weight-independent dosing of 25 to 30 mL, which usually is injected at 2 to 3 mL/s, followed by a saline flush at a similar rate. These have led to an increase in SNR/CNR that can support the recommended higher spatial resolutions on first-pass CE MR angiograms in most patients who are imaged at 1.5T. Still, in some patients who have poor cardiac output or in whom the gadolinium bolus was not well timed, the IQ on the 50- to 60-second CE MR angiogram is not optimal. More SNR/CNR would be helpful in these patients.

Intracranial TOF MR angiography has benefited from the increased SNR/CNR at 3T, compared with 1.5T [29]. There is the expectation that the same will be true for extracranial carotid MR angiography at 3T. Extension of extracranial carotid MR angiography to 3T has been limited by the lack of available eight-channel or higher neurovascular coils. While waiting for eight-channel 3T neurovascular coils to become available clinically, the authors have embarked on a project using dedicated 3T carotid surface coils to visualize the carotid bifurcation.

3T carotid contrast-enhanced MR angiography and plaque imaging using dedicated surface coils

There is extensive experience with dedicated carotid surface coils at 1.5T to visualize the carotid plaque at the level of the carotid bifurcation. The markedly improved SNR/CNR that is provided by these coils at 1.5T, compared with standard neurovascular coils, led some investigators to explore even higher resolution carotid CE MR angiography. The authors wished to extend this experience by using a modern short-bore 3T MR scanner combined with dedicated carotid surface coils to optimize carotid CE MR angiography of the carotid bifurcation and carotid plaque imaging.

Referring back to the article by Fain and colleagues [28]; one key factor in improving the performance of elliptic-centric phase reordered CE MR angiography as measured by the point-spread function (PSF) is to minimize the phase FOV in the y and z axes. By focusing on just the middle 14 to 16 cm of the neck, the phase FOV can be limited in both directions while generating substantially higher resolution CE MR angiography, compared with using a larger FOV and an eight-channel neurovascular coil. The improved performance from the dedicated carotid surface coils, as well as the 3T MR scanner, provides the necessary SNR/CNR to support this higher prescribed spatial resolution. The improved PSF that is provided by the smaller phase FOV should result in a sharper depiction of the arterial lumen boundary compared with a similar prescribed spatial resolution using a larger FOV. Stated another way, the same spatial resolution prescribed using a large FOV would result in inferior CE MR angiography compared with a small FOV because of the effect of the smaller phase FOV on the PSF. The arterial lumen boundaries would not be as sharp, despite the same prescribed resolution. This discussion also assumes that enough SNR/CNR is generated using the larger neurovascular coil. In addition to a small FOV in the x–y direction, less coverage in the z direction can be acquired by covering only the middle portion of the neck. Larger-phase FOV in the z direction is required to cover the entire course of the carotid artery from the arch through the circle of Willis. If even higher resolution carotid CE MR angiography is required, Fain and colleagues [28] predicted that a small-phase FOV in the y and z directions would be optimal.

Townsend and colleagues [7] demonstrated that swapping the phase and frequency directions (phase direction superior–inferior [SI]) with carotid CE MR angiography improved depiction of the lumen in their carotid stenosis model, using pulsatile flow. Because typical large FOV CE MR angiography acquisitions require the frequency direction to be SI, it has not been possible to swap phase and frequency. With the dedicated carotid coil imaging only the center portion of the neck with a 14- to 16-cm FOV CE MR angiography, this limitation is lifted. Therefore, the authors also have used a frequency direction of right to left, and phase-encoding gradients in the SI and AP directions. The natural signal drop-out of the four-channel surface coil, which consists of a pair of coils overlapped in the AP direction, limits problems with phase wrap in the SI direction.

Initial clinical experience with 500- to 600-μm carotid contrast-enhanced MR angiography at 3T

The authors' clinical protocol combines these above ideas by using a modern short-bore 3T MR with high performance gradients (40 mTm) and a four-channel dedicated carotid surface coil. The imaging parameters of repetition time (TR)/echo time (TE)/flip angle/number of excitations (NEX) are 5.7/1.3/30°/1. We prescribe an oblique 3.2-cm thick coronal slab of 14 to 16 cm with a 256 × 256 matrix, and use 40 partitions, each of which is 0.8 mm in thickness. The scan time is 59 seconds. Based upon an FOV of 15 cm, which is the authors' standard technique, the prescribed resolution of this 3T CE MR angiogram is 0.59 × 0.59 × 0.8 mm before zero-filling. This corresponds to a voxel volume of 0.27 mm^3, compared with 0.66 mm^3 as used by Willinek and colleagues [8], at 1.5T using a neurovascular coil. Zero-interpolation is used in all three directions, which results in a voxel volume of 0.03 mm^3. We also use a double dose of Gd-BOPTA (Multihance [Bracco, Princeton, New Jersey]) to improve the SNR/CNR. A routine timing dose study is performed first with 1 mL of Gd-BOPTA.

In the authors' first 15 patients, all 500- to 600-μm carotid CE MR angiograms demonstrated good to excellent intra-arterial contrast with little or no venous contamination. There was mild motion artifact on only one patient. In three cases so far, we have had DSA correlation. Fig. 1 demonstrates the excellent agreement between the 500- to 600-μm carotid CE MR angiography and the DSA. On the left, the internal carotid artery was measured as having a 78% stenosis by NASCET criteria, and was measured as having an 80% stenosis on the DSA by two observers without knowledge of the other study. Fig. 2 illustrates another severe narrowing which measured 70% by NASCET criteria. Notice the detail of the luminal surface and distinction of the edge of the vessel provided by the 500- to 600-μm carotid CE MR angiogram. Other examples of enhanced lumen depiction included the ability to depict a complex spiraling or corkscrew course of the patent internal carotid artery through the plaque at the level of the bulb, subtle shallow ulcers, and deep larger ulcerations. The high-resolution CE MR angiogram with 0.27 mm^3 voxel volume results in reducing T2* signal loss in regions of rapid susceptibility variation as discussed originally by Bernstein. There was little image distortion on the carotid CE MR angiogram, despite the presence of multiple surgical clips in two patients.

The sharp appearance of the carotid lumen walls on the CE MR angiogram is due to three factors. First, the prescribed resolution is the highest that has been reported for in vivo carotid CE MR angiography. This represents a 60% reduction in voxel volume compared with previous work by Willinek and colleagues [8]. There is less partial volume averaging with the increased spatial resolution. This increased resolution is a step closer to the 300-μm resolution of 3D rotational DSA. Secondly, we used

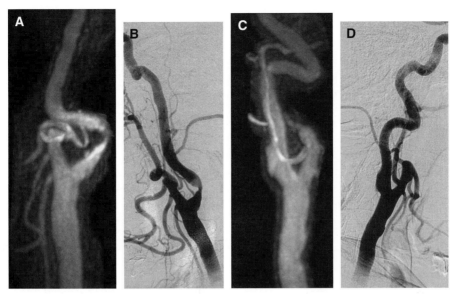

Figure 1 580 μm in-plane resolution 3T carotid CE MR angiogram (MRA) compared with selective DSA. (*A*) Maximum-intensity projection of 3T CE MRA demonstrates a severe narrowing of the proximal left internal carotid artery calculated to measure 78% diameter stenosis. (*B*) Corresponding selective DSA of the left carotid bifurcation confirms the severe (80%) stenosis. (*C*) Plaque at the right carotid bifurcation is causing less than a 30% diameter stenosis as seen on this maximum-intensity projection of 3T CE MRA. (*D*) This finding is confirmed on the selective right carotid bifurcation DSA.

the increased SNR/CNR from 3T, along with the improved efficiency of dedicated carotid surface coil and a double dose of a higher relaxtivity gadolinium agent (Gd BOPTA), to provide the necessary extra signal in an effort to ensure consistent IQ over a variety of patients. Lastly, the small FOV in the y and z directions is predicted to improve the sharpness of the lumen boundaries, according to the modeling of the PSF. Direct comparison of standard 1-mm resolution, large FOV carotid CE MR angiography with this new targeted small FOV 500- to 600-μm resolution carotid CE MR angiography, using DSA as the gold standard, is pending.

Initial clinical experience with carotid plaque imaging in vivo at 3T

In an effort to find more clinically relevant markers of plaque vulnerability, several noninvasive imaging strategies that use US, CT, and MR imaging have to be investigated. Of all these techniques, MR imaging shows the most promise for imaging the artery lumen, and at the same time, providing detailed information about the artery wall [30]. In 1996, Toussaint and coworkers [31] were among the first to demonstrate that 1.5T MR imaging is able to differentiate lipid core, fibrous cap, calcifications, and intraplaque hemorrhage, using T2-weighted images. By combining different MR imaging weightings, Shinnar and colleagues [32]

established that multisequence MR imaging is capable of identifying different plaque components with high sensitivity, specificity, and accuracy ex vivo. Subsequently, this work was extended to in vivo imaging. Hatsukami and colleagues [33] and Mitsumori and colleagues [34] demonstrated the ability of in vivo 1.5T MR imaging to depict ruptured fibrous cap with histologic correlation. Trivedi and colleagues [35] stressed the importance of this histologic marker to identify vulnerable carotid plaques. In vivo plaque imaging at 1.5T showed that soft plaque (necrotic core or hemorrhage) could be identified with 85% sensitivity and 92% specificity [36].

Recently, CE carotid plaque imaging at 1.5T was shown to be useful for improving plaque characterization [37,38]. There is better differentiation of the necrotic core from fibrous tissue when comparing pre- and postcontrast T1-weighted images. The postcontrast T1-weighted images have twice the SNR of other sequences to identify the necrotic core. These same images demonstrate that the degree of enhancement of fibrous regions relates to the amount of neovascularity [39]. Neovascularity is a key pathway for inflammatory cell infiltration. CE MR angiography demonstrates ulcerations better than does noncontrast TOF MR angiography [18]. The presence of ulcerations on invasive DSA [40] and carotid endarterectomy specimens [41] is associated with signs of plaque instability, such as

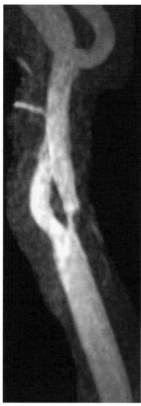

Figure 2 Right proximal internal carotid artery demonstrates a mildly irregular narrowing calculated to measure 71% diameter stenosis on this 580-μm in-plane resolution 3T carotid CE MR angiogram.

plaque rupture, intraplaque hemorrhage, and large lipid core. The improved detection of ulcerations on high-resolution CE MR angiography as proposed in this study offers greater sensitivity for identification of plaque instability.

Juxtaluminal calcifications are identified easily on bright-blood T1-weighted images from 3D TOF images using a 1.5T-MR scanner [42]. Kampschulte and colleagues' [43] study on carotid plaque hemorrhage suggested that juxtaluminal calcifications may be a causative factor of fibrous cap disruption and ulceration that lead to plaque instability. Juxtaluminal hemorrhage also was associated with these calcifications. The significance of intraplaque hemorrhage distant from the lumen and associated with an intact fibrous cap is less certain. Moody and colleagues [44] used a 1.5T MR scanner and reported that a specific T1-weighed sequence could differentiate between stable and unstable plaque by detecting high signal intensity within the plaque representing methemoglobin, an intermediate breakdown product of hemorrhage. Chu and colleagues [42] also identified intraplaque hemorrhage with high sensitivity (90%),

but with moderate specificity (74%). If the area of hemorrhage was large (>0.3 mm^2) or medium (0.1–0.3 mm^2) in size and was not associated with calcifications, there was much higher agreement between readers and with histology.

The authors believe that 3T MR imaging characterization of carotid plaque will be superior to 1.5T-MR imaging, primarily because of the increased SNR that is offered at 3T. Initial work on coronary plaque imaging at 3T showed a marked improvement in SNR and resulting IQ, compared with 1.5T [45]. Similar improvement in carotid plaque MR imaging at 3T was hypothesized. This is important because a large number of patients are excluded in current plaque studies at 1.5T as a result of poor IQ from poor SNR. In a recent assessment of multicontrast plaque imaging at 1.5T that was published in 2005, 18% to 35% of the patients were excluded because of poor IQ [46,47]. The authors decided to use similar slice thickness and in-plane resolution during their 3T MR carotid plaque imaging as are used in current 1.5T MR protocols. The achieved increase in SNR at 3T resulted in none of the first 15 patients being excluded from analysis because of poor IQ.

With the collaboration of the Vascular Imaging Laboratory at the University of Washington, the authors have modified the previously described black-blood T2 and T1 sequences that use double and quadruple inversion pulses, respectively [48,49]. The inversion times have been modified slightly to take into account the different T1 values at 3T compared with 1.5T. The imaging parameters are listed in Table 1. Please note the time efficiency of these sequences. Only 4 to 5 minutes are required for each type of contrast to image 36 mm of the plaque with 18 slices that are 2-mm thick. The entire plaque characterization using these four sequences (bright-blood T1-weighted images, black-blood T2-weighted images, black-blood T1-weighted images pre- and post-contrast) at 3T takes only 20 minutes of imaging time. Combined with the 500- to 600-μm carotid CE MR angiogram, the entire imaging study can be completed within 40 minutes. When new coils that can combine the characteristics of dedicated carotid bifurcation surface coils and the large FOV coverage of current neurovascular coils are available at 3T, it should be possible to combine an additional CE MR angiogram to cover the entire course of the carotid arteries from the aortic arch to the skull base with a 3D MOTSA (multiple overlapping thin slab angiography) MR angiogram of the intracranial vessels and limited FLAIR (fluid attenuation inversion recovery), T2-weighted image, and diffusion axial images of the brain into a comprehensive examination.

The appearance of various carotid plaque components was described at 1.5T and is listed in Table 2

Table 1: **Summary of imaging parameters for 3T carotid MR angiography and plaque imaging using dedicated carotid surface coils**

		Sequence			
Parameters	3D TOF	Black-blood DIR T2WI	Black-blood QIR T1WI	First-pass CE MRA	Black-blood QIR T1WI
TR (ms)	20–30	4000	800	5–6	800
TE (ms)	3–4	50	9–11	1.2–1.4	9–11
TI (ms)		240	520		520
FOV (cm)	16	16	16	15	16
Matrix	256 × 256	256 × 256	256 × 256	256 × 256	256 × 256
Resolution[a] (mm^2)	0.625 × 0.625	0.625 × 0.62	0.625 × 0.625	0.58 × 0.58	0.625 × 0.625
Thickness/spacing[b] (mm)	1/−0.5	2/0	2/0	0.8/0.4	2/0
Number of slices	40	18	18	40	18
Time (min)	4:00	4:32	5:18	0:59	5:18

Abbreviations: DIR, double inversion recovery; MRA, MR angiogram; QIR, quadruple inversion pulse; T1WI, T1-weighted image; T2WI, T2-weighted image.
[a] Resolution before interpolation, all images interpolated to 512 × 512.
[b] 3D series interpolated in z direction and overlapped by 50%, two-dimensional series are interleaved.

[46]. Initial experience indicates that the carotid plaque has similar characteristics at 3T. The identification of the lipid-rich necrotic core has been simplified greatly by relying upon the pre- and postcontrast T1-weighted images. The key is using the quadruple inversion pulse (QIR) sequence, which results in good blood suppression over a wide range of T1 values. Thus, the same QIR T1-weighted sequence can be used on the pre- and postcontrast images. This facilitates direct comparison and clearly shows the lipid-rich necrotic core as a region that does not enhance, and thus, appears dark on the postcontrast T1-weighted images. The lipid-rich necrotic core can be complicated by intraplaque hemorrhage. Depending upon its age, the hemorrhage can have a variety of appearances on the T1- and T2-weighted images [35]. This can complicate plaque characterization. On the postcontrast QIR T1-weighted images, most of the other plaque

components take on uniform signal intensity, which makes it easier to identify the dark lipid-rich necrotic core, even if it is associated with hemorrhage. Loose connective tissue is believed to represent areas of reparative process that could become vulnerable to ulceration. These are identified as high signal intensity on T2-weighted images and isointense to muscle on T1-weighted images. Plaque hemorrhage has a variety of signal characteristics, depending upon its age; however, it is easiest to identify as high signal intensity on the bright-blood T1-weighted image (source images from 3D TOF MR angiography). When hemorrhage is adjacent to the carotid lumen or associated with fibrous cap rupture, there may be an increased risk of thromboembolic disease to the brain. Juxtaluminal calcifications are seen easily as focal, well-defined regions of marked decrease signal intensity on the same bright-blood T1-weighted image.

Fig. 3 illustrates the typical IQ that the authors have achieved using the above in vivo carotid plaque protocol at 3T. Despite the severe stenosis that is seen on the CE MR angiogram, the carotid plaque is composed mostly of dense fibrous tissue that has signal characteristics that are similar to the adjacent sternocleidomastoid muscle on T1- and T2-weighted images. There is only a small area of loose connective tissue adjacent to the posterior lateral wall of the internal carotid artery lumen seen as a focal area of increased signal intensity on the T2-weighted images. No well-defined nonenhancing regions with the carotid plaque are identified on the postcontrast T1-weighted images to suggest a lipid-rich necrotic core. This benign-appearing plaque is completely different from the plaque that was seen in another patient who had a similarly appearing severe carotid stenosis. This is illustrated in Fig. 4, which shows a large

Table 2: **Carotid plaque classification criteria**

	TOF	T1W	PDW	T2W
Lipid rich necrotic core with				
No or little hemorrhage	0	0/+	0/+	−/0
Fresh hemorrhage	+	+	−/0	−/0
Recent hemorrhage	+	+	+	+
Calcification	−	−	−	−
Loose matrix	0	−/0	+	+
Dense (fibrous) tissue	−	0	0	0

The classification into subgroups is based on the following signal intensities relative to adjacent muscle. +, hyperintense; 0, isointense; −, hypointense.
Abbreviations: PDW, proton density weighted; T1W, T1 weighted; T2W, T2 weighted.

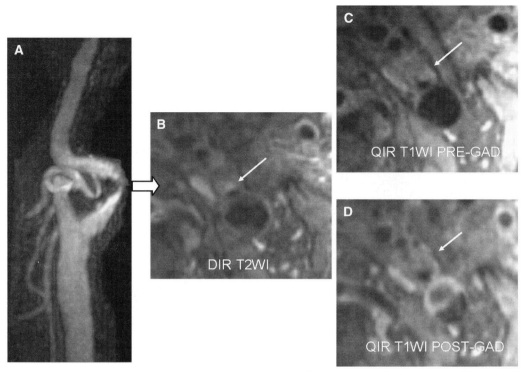

Figure 3 Severe carotid stenosis is associated with mostly dense fibrous tissue carotid plaque. (*A*) Maximum-intensity projection of 3T CE MR angiogram demonstrates a severe narrowing of the proximal left internal carotid artery calculated to measure 78% diameter stenosis. (*B*) Black-blood T2-weighted image (T2WI) demonstrates a small region that is hyperintense to surrounding muscle and is compatible with loose matrix (*arrow*). DIR, double inversion recovery. (*C*) Precontrast black-blood T1-weighted image (T1WI) reveals a homogenous plaque that is isointense to surrounding muscle which is compatible with a plaque that is mostly dense fibrous tissue (*arrow*). (*D*) Postcontrast black-blood T1-weighted image does not demonstrate any nonenhancing regions to suggest a lipid-rich necrotic core (*arrow*).

lipid-rich necrotic core. The size of the lipid core may be an important determinant of plaque instability [38]. Ouhlous and colleagues [45] identified the lipid core in 25 of 41 patients who had symptomatic severe carotid artery stenosis and were scheduled for carotid endarterectomy. Patients who have a lipid core have an ipsilateral infarct noted on brain MR imaging more often than do patients who do not have a lipid core (68% versus 31%, *P* = .03). They concluded that plaque composition as assessed by noncontrast MR imaging is related to the presence and extent of ischemic cerebral lesions. The presence of this more complex, possibly more dangerous, plaque cannot be predicted from the carotid CE MR angiogram alone. Thus, the authors believe that the addition of carotid plaque imaging at 3T to the 500- to 600-μm resolution CE MR angiogram may help to identify patients who are at increased risk for thromboembolic disease. This subset of patients may benefit from closer clinical monitoring, more aggressive medical therapy (eg, high-dose statin therapy), or even surgical intervention. The optimal treatment scheme awaits prospective longitudinal studies of carotid plaque morphology to determine better the natural history of the various plaque components that can be identified at 3T.

Initial clinical experience with large field-of-view carotid contrast-enhanced MR angiography at 3T

Initially, adaptation of large FOV carotid CE MR angiography at 3T was limited by the lack of high-quality neurovascular coils to image the entire course of the carotid artery from the aortic arch through the circle of Willis. All major MR manufacturers now provide eight-channel or higher neurovascular coils for 3T scanners. When converting protocols from 1.5T to 3T, several factors need to be taken into consideration. Chemical shift and susceptibility variation double when measured in Hertz as the field strength increases. Typically, receiver bandwidth is increased for a 3T protocol compared with 1.5T. At 3T, the echo time at which fat and water have opposed phase for gradient echo imaging are different than at 1.5T (TE = 1.2

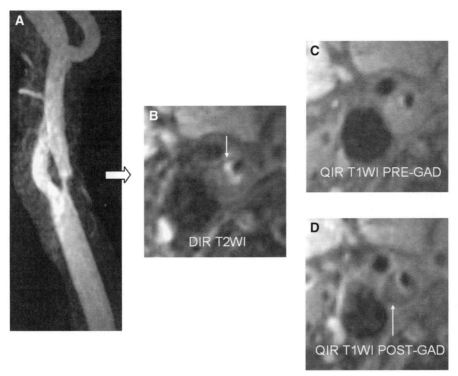

Figure 4 Complex appearing plaque is noted in a different patient who had severe carotid stenosis. (*A*) Maximum-intensity projection of 3T CE MR angiogram demonstrates a severe narrowing of the proximal left internal carotid artery calculated to measure 71% diameter stenosis. (*B*) Black-blood T2-weighted image (T2WI) demonstrates a region next to the internal carotid artery lumen that is hyperintense to surrounding muscle (*arrow*) and is compatible with loose matrix. Most of the remainder of the plaque is hypointense to muscle, which suggests a large lipid-rich necrotic core. DIR, double inversion recovery. (*C, D*) By comparing the black-blood T1-weighted images (T1WI) before (*C*) and after contrast (*D*), a large nonenhancing region (*arrow*) that occupies more than 50% of the cross-sectional area of the carotid plaque can be appreciated. This corresponds to a large, lipid-rich necrotic core.

milliseconds, 3.5 milliseconds, 5.8 milliseconds for fat/water out-of-phase at 3T). Specific absorption rate (SAR) quadruples at 3T compared with 1.5T. As a result, the regulatory limits for SAR are reached more quickly at 3T and have been a limitation for 3T MR angiography. Because the radiofrequency (RF) power deposited is proportional to the square of the flip angle, reducing it by a few degrees decreases the RF power deposition to within acceptable limits for 3T carotid CE MR angiography.

For comparable geometry RF coils, the SNR at 3T approximately doubles compared with 1.5T. Some recommended protocols for large-FOV carotid CE MR angiograms are listed in Table 3. Note that the voxel volumes are 25% to 40% less than those that typically are used at 1.5T. Although they do not equal the voxel volumes that have been reached by using dedicated carotid surface coils, these sequences provide excellent coverage of the entire course of the carotid artery from the aortic arch through the skull base. The decreased voxel volume also decreases T2* signal loss at the skull base.

Table 3: Recommended protocol for 3T carotid first-pass three-dimensional elliptic-centric contrast-enhanced MR angiography

TR (ms)	5–6 (minimum)
TE (ms)	1.4–1.6 (minimum)
FOVx (cm)	24–26
FOVy (cm)	16–18
Matrix	
Frequency	384–512
Phase	256–288
Resolution[a] (mm^2)	0.54 × 0.83
Thickness/spacing[b] (mm)	1.2/−0.6
Number of slices	50
Time (min)	0:55–1:10

[a] Resolution before interpolation assuming 24-cm FOV with 448 × 288 matrix, all images interpolated to 512 × 512.
[b] 3D series interpolated in z direction and overlapped by 50%.

Initial clinical experience indicates that there is an observable increase in SNR/CNR with the carotid CE MR angiography at 3T using the 8-channel neurovascular coils, although it is not a true doubling. This is due, in part, to the fact that not all tissues achieve a true doubling of SNR when moving from 1.5T to 3T. CE MR angiogram parameters, such as flip angle, TR, TE, and bandwidth, as well as optimal eight-channel or higher coil designs will impact the final observable increase in SNR/CNR. Improved IQ of carotid CE MR angiography at 3T with higher resolution and SNR/CNR, compared with 1.5T, is evident (Fig. 5). The bottom line is that with the availability of new eight-channel neurovascular coils, carotid CE MR angiography is easier at 3T scanning than at 1.5T scanning.

Summary

Some controversy exists over the accuracy and optimal parameters for carotid CE MR angiography at 1.5T. Spatial resolution remains more important than does temporal resolution to address the key question of vessel stenosis, based upon a review of the available literature that compares CE MR angiography with DSA. Specifically, CE MR angiograms with 0.9- to 1.2-mm resolution in all three planes before interpolation have a high reported sensitivity and specificity compared with DSA. To achieve this type of spatial resolution, cover the entire course of the carotid arteries from the aortic arch through the skull base, and achieve an absence of venous signal usually requires an elliptic-centric phase encoding CE MR angiogram that lasts for 50 to 60 seconds without the use of parallel imaging techniques. This near-millimeter resolution requires an accurate timing of the gadolinium bolus arrival to maximize intra-arterial SNR and to minimize venous contamination. Parallel imaging techniques can decrease the imaging time, but at a cost of some SNR. Initial experience with eight-channel or higher neurovascular coils at 3T indicates an increase in SNR/CNR compared with 1.5T. This should allow more consistent submillimeter-resolution carotid CE MR angiography with adequate SNR to maintain good IQ in a wide variety of clinical patients. Although a definite, prospective comparison of various CE MR angiography techniques, including a 20- to 30-second scan with 1.2- to 1.4-mm^3 voxel resolution and 50- to 60-second scan with 0.9- to 1.1-mm^3 voxel resolution at 1.5T, as well as 0.5- to 0.6-mm^3 voxel resolution with scan time of 50 to 60 seconds at 3T versus rotational DSA does not exist, the expectation is that the higher resolution and increased SNR that has resulted from 3T carotid CE MR angiography will have high sensitivity and specificity in detecting severe carotid stenosis.

The most exciting application of 3T for carotid artery imaging may not be the higher resolution CE MR angiogram, however. Early work has demonstrated the potential of 3T, combined with sensitive

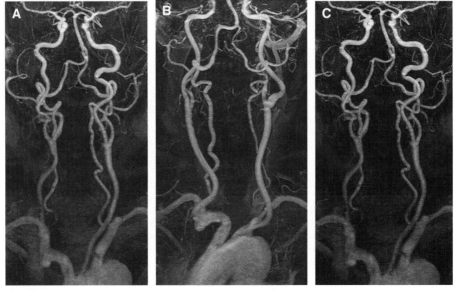

Figure 5 Three examples of 3T carotid CE MR angiography using a new eight-channel neurovascular coil. Note the good to excellent ultra-arterial filling with little or no venous contamination. The arterial lumen edge is well defined because of the submillimeter in-plane resolution.

surface coils, to depict carotid plaque with sufficient SNR to identify important plaque components consistently in most patients. This could help move MR imaging of the carotid arteries away from a strict evaluation of luminal narrowing to a focused evaluation of plaque morphology. Much work needs to be done. Although there is a growing body of literature to support the contention that plaque morphology is a predictor of subsequent thromboembolic disease, the natural history of these various plaque components in a large number of patients needs to be elucidated. If plaque characterization proves to be an independent risk factor that predicts stroke, more aggressive clinical treatment option strategies may be devised for patients who are at the highest risk. Currently, plaque characterization at 3T requires a different set of coils compared with the global assessment of the entire course of the carotid arteries. Future generations of 16- to 32-channel carotid coils should be able to combine the best features of current 4- to 8-channel surface carotid coils and neurovascular coils. These will enable a comprehensive evaluation of the entire course of the carotid artery and detailed carotid bifurcation plaque characterization at 3T within a clinically acceptable 1-hour time frame. This comprehensive carotid artery evaluation with 3T MR imaging would be far superior to that which is possible with US or CT.

References

[1] Beneficial effect of carotid endarterectomy in symptomatic patients with high-grade carotid stenosis. North American Symptomatic Carotid Endarterectomy Trial Collaborators. N Engl J Med 1991;325:445–53.

[2] Randomised trial of endarterectomy for recently symptomatic carotid stenosis: final results of the MRC European Carotid Surgery Trial (ECST). Lancet 1998;351:1379–87.

[3] Rothwell PM, Eliasziw M, Gutnikov SA, et al. Analysis of pooled data from the randomised controlled trials of endarterectomy for symptomatic carotid stenosis. Lancet 2003;361:107–16.

[4] Anderson CM, Lee RE, Levin DL, et al. Measurement of internal carotid artery stenosis from source MR angiograms. Radiology 1994;193:219–26.

[5] Kent KC, Kuntz KM, Patel MR, et al. Perioperative imaging strategies for carotid endarterectomy. An analysis of morbidity and cost-effectiveness in symptomatic patients. JAMA 1995;274:888–93.

[6] Patel MR, Kuntz KM, Klufas RA, et al. Preoperative assessment of the carotid bifurcation. Can magnetic resonance angiography and duplex ultrasonography replace contrast arteriography? Stroke 1995;26:1753–8.

[7] Townsend TC, Saloner D, Pan XM, et al. Contrast material-enhanced MRA overestimates severity of carotid stenosis, compared with 3D time-of-flight MRA. J Vasc Surg 2003;38:36–40.

[8] Willinek WA, von Falkenhausen M, Born M, et al. Noninvasive detection of steno-occlusive disease of the supra-aortic arteries with three-dimensional contrast-enhanced magnetic resonance angiography: a prospective, intra-individual comparative analysis with digital subtraction angiography. Stroke 2005;36:38–43.

[9] Fellner C, Lang W, Janka R, et al. Magnetic resonance angiography of the carotid arteries using three different techniques: accuracy compared with intraarterial x-ray angiography and endarterectomy specimens. J Magn Reson Imaging 2005;21:424–31.

[10] Alvarez-Linera J, Benito-Leon J, Escribano J, et al. Prospective evaluation of carotid artery stenosis: elliptic centric contrast-enhanced MR angiography and spiral CT angiography compared with digital subtraction angiography. AJNR Am J Neuroradiol 2003;24:1012–9.

[11] Anzalone N, Scomazzoni F, Castellano R, et al. Carotid artery stenosis: intraindividual correlations of 3D time-of-flight MR angiography, contrast-enhanced MR angiography, conventional DSA, and rotational angiography for detection and grading. Radiology 2005;236:204–13.

[12] Aschenbach R, Eger C, Basche S, et al. [Grading of carotid artery stenosis using high resolution dynamic magnetic resonance angiography in comparison to intraarterial digital subtraction angiography. Are stenoses over 70% reliably detectable?] Rofo 2004;176:357–62.

[13] Borisch I, Horn M, Butz B, et al. Preoperative evaluation of carotid artery stenosis: comparison of contrast-enhanced MR angiography and duplex sonography with digital subtraction angiography. AJNR Am J Neuroradiol 2003;24:1117–22.

[14] Butz B, Dorenbeck U, Borisch I, et al. High-resolution contrast-enhanced magnetic resonance angiography of the carotid arteries using fluoroscopic monitoring of contrast arrival: diagnostic accuracy and interobserver variability. Acta Radiol 2004;45:164–70.

[15] Cosottini M, Pingitore A, Puglioli M, et al. Contrast-enhanced three-dimensional magnetic resonance angiography of atherosclerotic internal carotid stenosis as the noninvasive imaging modality in revascularization decision making. Stroke 2003;34:660–4.

[16] Goyal M, Nicol J, Gandhi D. Evaluation of carotid artery stenosis: contrast-enhanced magnetic resonance angiography compared with conventional digital subtraction angiography. Can Assoc Radiol J 2004;55:111–9.

[17] Hathout GM, Duh MJ, El-Saden SM. Accuracy of contrast-enhanced MR angiography in predicting angiographic stenosis of the internal carotid artery: linear regression analysis. AJNR Am J Neuroradiol 2003;24:1747–56.

[18] Huston III J, Fain SB, Wald JT, et al. Carotid artery: elliptic centric contrast-enhanced MR angiography compared with conventional angiography. Radiology 2001;218:138–43.

[19] Johnston DC, Goldstein LB. Clinical carotid endarterectomy decision making: noninvasive vascular imaging versus angiography. Neurology 2001;56:1009–15.

[20] Lenhart M, Framme N, Volk M, et al. Time-resolved contrast-enhanced magnetic resonance angiography of the carotid arteries: diagnostic accuracy and inter-observer variability compared with selective catheter angiography. Invest Radiol 2002;37:535–41.

[21] Nederkoorn PJ, Elgersma OE, van der Graaf Y, et al. Carotid artery stenosis: accuracy of contrast-enhanced MR angiography for diagnosis. Radiology 2003;228:677–82.

[22] Randoux B, Marro B, Koskas F, et al. Carotid artery stenosis: prospective comparison of CT, three-dimensional gadolinium-enhanced MR, and conventional angiography. Radiology 2001; 220:179–85.

[23] Remonda L, Senn P, Barth A, et al. Contrast-enhanced 3D MR angiography of the carotid artery: comparison with conventional digital subtraction angiography. AJNR Am J Neuroradiol 2002;23:213–9.

[24] Sundgren PC, Sunden P, Lindgren A, et al. Carotid artery stenosis: contrast-enhanced MR angiography with two different scan times compared with digital subtraction angiography. Neuroradiology 2002;44:592–9.

[25] U-King-Im J, Trivedi RA, Graves MJ, et al. Contrast-enhanced MR angiography for carotid disease: diagnostic and potential clinical impact. Neurology 2004;62:1282–90.

[26] Wutke R, Lang W, Fellner C, et al. High-resolution, contrast-enhanced magnetic resonance angiography with elliptical centric k-space ordering of supra-aortic arteries compared with selective X-ray angiography. Stroke 2002;33:1522–9.

[27] Yang CW, Carr JC, Futterer SF, et al. Contrast-enhanced MR angiography of the carotid and vertebrobasilar circulations. AJNR Am J Neuroradiol 2005;26:2095–101.

[28] Fain SB, Riederer SJ, Bernstein MA, et al. Theoretical limits of spatial resolution in elliptical-centric contrast-enhanced 3D-MRA. Magn Reson Med 1999;42:1106–16.

[29] Bernstein MA, Huston III J, Lin C, et al. High-resolution intracranial and cervical MRA at 3.0T: technical considerations and initial experience. Magn Reson Med 2001;46:955–62.

[30] Yuan C, Kerwin WS. MRI of atherosclerosis. J Magn Reson Imaging 2004;19:710–9.

[31] Toussaint JF, LaMuraglia GM, Southern JF, et al. Magnetic resonance images lipid, fibrous, calcified, hemorrhagic, and thrombotic components of human atherosclerosis in vivo. Circulation 1996;94:932–8.

[32] Shinnar M, Fallon JT, Wehrli S, et al. The diagnostic accuracy of ex vivo MRI for human atherosclerotic plaque characterization. Arterioscler Thromb Vasc Biol 1999;19:2756–61.

[33] Hatsukami TS, Ross R, Polissar NL, et al. Visualization of fibrous cap thickness and rupture in human atherosclerotic carotid plaque in vivo with high-resolution magnetic resonance imaging. Circulation 2000;102:959–64.

[34] Mitsumori LM, Hatsukami TS, Ferguson MS, et al. In vivo accuracy of multisequence MR imaging for identifying unstable fibrous caps in advanced human carotid plaques. J Magn Reson Imaging 2003;17:410–20.

[35] Trivedi RA, U-King-Im J, Graves MJ, et al. MRI-derived measurements of fibrous-cap and lipid-core thickness: the potential for identifying vulnerable carotid plaques in vivo. Neuroradiology 2004;46:738–43.

[36] Yuan C, Mitsumori LM, Ferguson MS, et al. In vivo accuracy of multispectral magnetic resonance imaging for identifying lipid-rich necrotic cores and intraplaque hemorrhage in advanced human carotid plaques. Circulation 2001; 104:2051–6.

[37] Wasserman BA, Smith WI, Trout III HH, et al. Carotid artery atherosclerosis: in vivo morphologic characterization with gadolinium-enhanced double-oblique MR imaging initial results. Radiology 2002;223:566–73.

[38] Yuan C, Mitsumori LM, Beach KW, et al. Carotid atherosclerotic plaque: noninvasive MR characterization and identification of vulnerable lesions. Radiology 2001;221:285–99.

[39] Yuan C, Kerwin WS, Ferguson MS, et al. Contrast-enhanced high resolution MRI for atherosclerotic carotid artery tissue characterization. J Magn Reson Imaging 2002;15:62–7.

[40] Lovett JK, Gallagher PJ, Hands LJ, et al. Histological correlates of carotid plaque surface morphology on lumen contrast imaging. Circulation 2004;110:2190–7.

[41] Fisher M, Paganini-Hill A, Martin A, et al. Carotid plaque pathology: thrombosis, ulceration, and stroke pathogenesis. Stroke 2005;36: 253–7.

[42] Chu B, Kampschulte A, Ferguson MS, et al. Hemorrhage in the atherosclerotic carotid plaque: a high-resolution MRI study. Stroke 2004; 35:1079–84.

[43] Kampschulte A, Ferguson MS, Kerwin WS, et al. Differentiation of intraplaque versus juxtaluminal hemorrhage/thrombus in advanced human carotid atherosclerotic lesions by in vivo magnetic resonance imaging. Circulation 2004; 110:3239–44.

[44] Moody AR, Murphy RE, Morgan PS, et al. Characterization of complicated carotid plaque with magnetic resonance direct thrombus imaging in patients with cerebral ischemia. Circulation 2003; 107:3047–52.

[45] Botnar RM, Stuber M, Lamerichs R, et al. Initial experiences with in vivo right coronary artery human MR vessel wall imaging at 3 tesla. J Cardiovasc Magn Reson 2003;5:589–94.

[46] Ouhlous M, Flack H, de Weert T, et al. Carotid plaque composition and cerebral infarction: MR imaging study. AJNR Am J Neuroradiol 2005;26:1044–9.

[47] Saam T, Ferguson MS, Yarnykh VL, et al. Quantitative evaluation of carotid plaque composition by in vivo MRI. Arterioscler Thromb Vasc Biol 2005;25:234–9.

[48] Yarnykh VL, Yuan C. Multislice double inversion-recovery black-blood imaging with simultaneous slice reinversion. J Magn Reson Imaging 2003;17:478–83.

[49] Yarnykh VL, Yuan C. T1-insensitive flow suppression using quadruple inversion-recovery. Magn Reson Med 2002;48:899–905.

ELSEVIER
SAUNDERS

MAGNETIC
RESONANCE
IMAGING CLINICS

Magn Reson Imaging Clin N Am (2006) 123–125

Index

Note: Page numbers of article titles are in **boldface** type.

Changing Your Address?

Make sure your subscription changes too! When you notify us of your new address, you can help make our job easier by including an exact copy of your Clinics label number with your old address (see illustration below.) This number identifies you to our computer system and will speed the processing of your address change. Please be sure this label number accompanies your old address and your corrected address—you can send an old Clinics label with your number on it or just copy it exactly and send it to the address listed below.

We appreciate your help in our attempt to give you continuous coverage. Thank you.

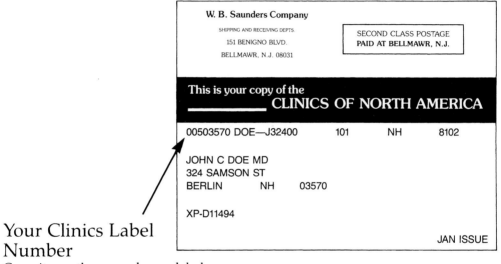

Your Clinics Label Number
Copy it exactly or send your label
along with your address to:
W.B. Saunders Company, Customer Service
Orlando, FL 32887-4800
Call Toll Free 1-800-654-2452

Please allow four to six weeks for delivery of new subscriptions and for processing address changes.